DRY FASTING REVOLUTION

THE PRACTICAL GUIDE

Editing, design, typesetting and publishing by UK Book Publishing

www.ukbookpublishing.com

ISBN: 978-1-917329-18-7

Foreword by Dr Chaligne

I had the extraordinary opportunity to meet Michel Deladoey and take part in a dry fasting retreat in Montenegro in 2020. The breathtakingly beautiful scenery provided the backdrop for a truly unique adventure. This retreat marked a turning point in my life, as it preceded an event I'd been hoping for, for a long time: the birth of my first child. At the age of 47, thanks to dry fasting, I was able to experience the benefits of deep cleansing and cellular regeneration, leading to this wonderful news.

Admittedly I'm no expert on the subject, but it's clear that dry fasting has the power to purify the body and revitalise every cell. Our dry fasting journey has been carefully guided to maximise the benefits of this practice. Despite challenges such as fatigue and thirst, we incorporated walks in the forest and sunrise ice water affusions into our routine. Every moment was precious.

I'm firmly convinced of the importance of being supported by professionals in this process. Complementary treatments such as massage, meditation, yoga and listening to music play a crucial role in reconciling body and mind, helping to dispel anxieties and negative thoughts.

I would like to express my deep gratitude to Michel for guiding me through this exceptional experience, which revealed to me the miracle of life: my child. Not only did this fast help me to regain my energy and serenity, it also helped me to balance my weight.

While I'm waiting to repeat this treatment at least twice a year, I'd like to continue restoring my metabolic and energy balance, particularly after breast-feeding.

With all my friendship,

Cristina Gabriela Chaligne, Doctor of Medicine

Foreword by Dr Raphaël Perez

I've known Michel for about two years and our exchanges have been very rich and not necessarily opposed as one might imagine between a specialist in dry fasting and a specialist in water fasting (hygienist).

Dry fasting is not in opposition to water fasting but rather a different way of approaching fasting. It is a way of putting the body into a different physiological state. More and more people are experimenting with fasting, and many try it without necessarily realising what it means for the body. Unfortunately, we are seeing the results of people having bad experiences. But also, fortunately many more people who come out of the experience in a very positive way.

Fasting is a natural practice, and one that we should all be able to carry out without any risk in a more or less restrictive (more or less advanced) way. But it is prepared and carried out correctly. The most common problems frequently encountered stem from an inappropriate approach to fasting. This is as true for water fasting as it is for dry fasting. But in the case of dry fasting, the context in which the fast is prepared and carried out is even more important.

The mind and the emotions are part of our being. These components are too often neglected in the context of fasting, just as they are in our daily lives.

Fasting has more than just physical effects. There are also mental and emotional effects. To ignore this is to say that we are only partially fasting. Fasting has a profound influence on our being. It can unblock and free us mentally and emotionally. And as things go in both directions, forgetting to take account of the mental and emotional aspects when preparing for and carrying out a fast can create blockages, making fasting less effective.

Michel's aim is to make dry fasting accessible to as many people as possible. But above all, to do it safely. This book 'The Dry Fasting Revolution: A Practical Guide' is very much part of this approach. It's not just another book about on fasting, rehashing what we've already read many times. Michel has succeeded in making this book a truly educational and accessible tool, and a guide to practising dry fasting with maximum safety. The mental and the emotional are two components that he has integrated into his dry fasting practice and which he passes on here.

This book is a very good guide for moving from theory to practice without unnecessary steps.

Raphaël Perez, Dr in pharmacy – naturopath
Director of a training organisation in naturopathy and fasting

Foreword by Thierry Casasnovas

I remember one day in the summer of 2015, when I was giving a course in the centre of France. We were at that part of the course where I was talking about fasting, its countless benefits, its limits and the precautions to be taken.

The question of water and dry fasting came up naturally, and as a good 'little parrot', repeating what my trainers had told me without having experienced it themselves, I warned against any form of fasting that banned water for more than 48 hours.

Too dangerous! The sentence was final...

On this course, there was an elderly lady whom we had all noticed.

Sabine.

There was something paradoxical about her: objectively, we recognised her great age. But her voice, her alertness, her physical flexibility and her dynamism were those of someone thirty years younger.

Halfway through my presentation, Sabine raised her hand to ask to speak.

She explained that in her life she had fasted several times without water or any other liquid, each for more than ten days, and that not only had she not died, but she had also witnessed some very significant healings after these fasts. Above all, she based all her extraordinary vitality on this regular practice of dry fasting.

Not without a touch of mischief, she looked me straight in the eye and asked: 'Have you tried it?

It has to be said that I had given up on the alarmist warnings from my naturopathic trainers.

His testimony deeply disturbed my beliefs. After this course, I set out to understand.

How could a body go through a period of several days without water without damage? What were the physiological mechanisms involved?

Once I understood, I experimented...

And as a result of my experiences, I now only fast dry, without water.

Water fasting and dry fasting are not opposites, as Dr Raphaël Perez wisely points out; they are two different experiences.

For my part, I really fell in love with the practice of dry fasting, to the point of devoting hours of videos to it in order to de-diabolise the practice.

I'm a lover of life, and it›s clear that never before have we been able to touch the incredible potential for life and healing that lies within each and every one of us as much as with dry fasting.

However, this unparalleled intensity demands that we don›t do just anything. Firstly, to reap all the benefits, but also to avoid hurting yourself and going beyond your limits.

I was already very enthusiastic when Michel Daladoey›s first book came out.

At the time, the only written material we had was a rough translation of a Russian work by Dr Filonov, which gave little information about the method.

This first book laid a solid, scientific foundation for understanding why dry fasting was so interesting.

What was missing was a practical guide, so that as many people as possible could experience dry fasting in complete safety.

I think I can say that this has now been done, brilliantly, without omitting all the dimensions of the being and the incredible challenge that dry fasting represents.

This holistic guide is a unique and essential book, the product of extremely solid experience and exemplary scientific rigour, designed to popularise the practice of dry fasting.

It's an honour for me to be able to preface it, and I can't thank Michel enough for his confidence in me.

Thierry Casasnovas
A passionate promoter of hygiene and naturopathy
Videographer and trainer

Introduction

In this innovative book, we explore the concept of holistic dry fasting, a comprehensive approach to improving health in a sustainable way. It is a unique and effective healing method that works on the root causes of pathologies. This book will guide you through concrete practices and provide you with simple tools to manage your dry fasting independently. It will equip you with the knowledge you need to understand your body's reactions and, above all, to avoid any danger. Modern dry fasting is presented as a method of introspective self-healing, seeking to maximise the physical, psychological and spiritual potential of the individual. It is inspired by ancestral common sense and the teachings common to all religions.

Although dry fasting is recognised as an effective means of self-cleansing, health maintenance and treatment, both in its short and prolonged forms, it is crucial never to lose sight of the importance of the terrain, as Hippocrates emphasised. This book, based on clinical practice and observations made during our cures, provides a comprehensive overview of the constantly evolving dry fasting method.

A few key phrases

> *"In the interior of the body there is an unknown agent that works for the whole and for the parts, which is both one and many, like the ants in an anthill that work individually on their tasks for the good of the whole".*
>
> **Hippocrates**

Although modern medicine has made considerable advances, it now seems to be reaching certain limits in terms of therapeutic effectiveness, focusing more on eliminating symptoms than on understanding the underlying causes of imbalances. As a result, it no longer fully meets the health and well-being needs of today's population. It is in a global and holistic approach, looking at care over the long term, that real prospects for healing are emerging. Active involvement in one's own healing process is a key element of health.

It is also essential to recognise our body's remarkable and often underestimated power of self-healing. Total trust in our body is crucial during the process of transformation and evolution that is illness. In this sense, dry fasting, which consists of allowing the body to rest without any external input, is an effective and powerful means of promoting self-healing.

Both animals and human beings have a genetic code designed to recycle, renew and regenerate anything superfluous or undesirable, a process known as autophagy, a unique and therapeutic mechanism inherent in fasting.

Michel Deladoey

"The doctor of the future won't be giving out drugs; he'll be teaching his patients how to look after their bodies, nutrition and the causes and prevention of disease".
Thomas A. Edison, inventor of the phonograph, 1903.

"It is nature that cures diseases. She herself finds the appropriate ways, without needing to be directed by our intelligence".
Hippocrates

"No health without good digestion. We are not what we eat, we are what we digest or rather assimilate".
Dr Yann *Rougier*

Table of contents

Disclaimer and Legal Protection Statement

This book on dry fasting is purely informational and aims to share knowledge about a discipline practised by various religions worldwide for millennia. The fasting and yoga retreats we offer in different countries do not substitute for medical care or visits to the doctor and are not related to any medical approach. These retreats aim at health prevention and well-being, and they also involve a deep personal and emotional journey.

Each participant joins freely and consciously and can leave the retreat at any time. A spirit of benevolence and group support is the guiding principle during these retreats. We do not encourage or force anyone to fast or practise yoga during these retreats. Everything is voluntary and measured.

The facilitators are not there to treat or cure any medical condition. We emphasize individual responsibility and autonomy for optimal health. Participants are encouraged to consult with their healthcare providers before undertaking any fasting or yoga practices to ensure they are suitable for their health conditions.

Legal Notice

The information presented in this book and during our retreats is not intended to diagnose, treat, cure, or prevent any disease. The content provided is for educational purposes only and should not be considered as medical advice. Always seek the advice of your physician or other qualified health providers with any questions you may have regarding a medical condition.

By participating in our retreats, individuals acknowledge that they are doing so voluntarily and at their own risk. We are not responsible for any adverse effects or consequences resulting from the use of any suggestions, preparations, or procedures described in this book or during the retreats.

Dry fasting requires competent supervision to avoid mistakes. In case of any incident, the author cannot be held responsible for anything. Each person undertakes dry fasting freely and consciously. We do not encourage anyone to undertake fasting without the advice of a healthcare professional.

Statement for Authorities

Our fasting and yoga retreats are designed to promote health and well-being through traditional practices that have been recognized across various cultures and religions for centuries. We operate with full transparency and respect for individual autonomy. We do not compete with conventional medicine but rather offer complementary approaches for those seeking alternative methods for personal growth and well-being.

We welcome open dialogue with health authorities and are committed to ensuring that our practices comply with all relevant regulations and standards. Our goal is to support individuals in their journey towards better health in a safe, respectful, and legally compliant manner.

Introduction

Following the enthusiastic reception of my first book on therapeutic dry fasting and the growing success of our fasting retreats, where participants from all over the world come to explore this transformative practice, I'm delighted to present the sequel. Whether it's to treat a medical condition, maintain your health, or push back your personal limits, dry fasting is an essential path for anyone who aspires to greater autonomy and less fear in the face of adversity – including the fear of dying of thirst.

This ancient practice has been brought up to date, and remains a pillar for maintaining good health and positively influencing our destiny, by harmonising our physical and subtle bodies. In this new volume, you will discover practical approaches and adjustments in the preparation of fasting, now designed to be sustainable and integrated as a dietary adjustment to life and no longer as a periodic constraint as some might think. This book will guide you through concrete practices and provide you with simple tools to manage your dry fast independently. It will equip you with the knowledge you need to understand your body's reactions and, above all, to avoid any danger.

I have enriched the post-fasting recovery method with innovations to maximise the therapeutic and regenerative benefits of dry fasting, while avoiding the pitfalls of carbohydrates and post-fasting blood sugar fluctuations. Dry fasting is presented here as a catalyst for homeostatic processes, an integrative practice that does not dissociate the physical, mental and spiritual bodies, as everything works in synergy.

Dry fasting should be seen as an exploration of the self, an initiatory pilgrimage towards greater inner knowledge. My own fasting experiences have been deeply enriched over the years, becoming more accomplished technically, spiritually and emotionally, thanks in particular to the collaboration of Marie Christine Thomas, who has brought lightness and balance to the unique group retreats I organise. We will continue to evolve, encouraging each faster to take full responsibility for his or her life, thoughts, food and consumption. Achieving optimal health well into old age means creating your own art of living, based on the desire and motivation to adopt healthy habits and leave behind what makes you weak.

Choosing to practise dry fasting should become as natural and conscious a gesture as regularly maintaining your car. Far from being a constraint, it's an act of respect for our bodies, which will repay us in kind. Join us in this health revolution, where every step towards fasting is a step towards rediscovering yourself. I hope that this version will give readers an extra boost and stimulate your interest in dry fasting, encouraging you to explore and adopt this beneficial practice.

How did I come to dry fasting?

My career began far from the paths of therapy. First as a police officer in Switzerland, then as a member of the international police force for the UN, nothing in my background predestined me to embrace a vocation as a therapist or to become a support for those fighting for their health. However, my path took an unexpected turn after being vaccinated against yellow fever. The effects, although mild, were irreversible, causing persistent symptoms that I have tried to alleviate all my life, leading to unforeseen complications.

My last deployment to Côte d'Ivoire with UNOCI marked the end of my humanitarian career but the beginning of my personal quest for healing. Memories of war zones, visits to local prisons and flagrant injustices affected me deeply and generated lasting post-traumatic stress. Among these memories, the image of a young child threatened with being burnt alive for a simple theft remains engraved in my mind. With my colleague, an officer from Niger, we intervened to save the child from an angry mob. This scene, among many others, brought me face to face with brutal realities, but also showed me some unforgettable faces of humanity.

Back in Switzerland on leave, I fell seriously ill. Misdiagnosed as a simple case of dengue fever, I endured days of acute suffering before undetected malaria was finally recognised. The illness confined me to bed, shaking with pain every night. As my condition deteriorated, I was rushed to hospital. It was a fight for survival that lasted for months and the convalescence stretched well over a year. This period of vulnerability prompted me to look for natural alternatives for my recovery, which eventually led me to naturopathy. I discovered that knowledge of these methods could offer invaluable autonomy in health management, a far cry from conventional treatments which were often limited to emergency treatment.

Then came Lyme disease, an ordeal that eroded my health even further. Suffering from erythema migrans dating back to 2001, I learned that I also had co-infections. That's when I heard about dry fasting. Sceptical at first, I asked someone who had been cured by this method and finally decided to try it in Russia. After three intensive cures, I regained the health I thought I'd lost. This personal transformation convinced me of the need to spread the word about this practice.

Today, I'm continuing to develop and perfect the dry fasting method, while accompanying others who want to discover it. My mission is to make the practice simple, safe and accessible to everyone. I would also like to stress that each individual is responsible for his or her own healing journey. It is essential to understand that subconscious dynamics come into play during therapeutic dry fasting, phenomena that even a coach specialising in dry fasting cannot anticipate. The therapeutic dry fasting coach is not a healer and cannot be held responsible for any changes or incidents that occur during the fast. The fasting person must be prepared to embrace and accept all the experiences that may arise, whether they are pleasant or difficult.

Although short fasts can offer immediate benefits, long fasts tend to produce deeper and more lasting results. Despite a lack of recognition in traditional medical circles, I am convinced on the basis of empirical evidence that dry fasting, when practised correctly, can bring about remarkable transformations. I cherish the dream that one day the medical profession will study this method seriously and recognise its therapeutic potential, thus revealing the full extent of its benefits.

CHAPTER 1

Hygienism

1. A few notions of hygiene, a basic foundation for good health

Hygienism, as a system of thought and as a way of life, is based on profound foundations designed to promote holistic health through thoughtful lifestyle choices. Underpinning this philosophy is a fundamental belief in the body's inherent ability to maintain balance and heal itself when optimal conditions are created. By embracing this idea, hygienism places the emphasis on preventing illness rather than treating it, in a proactive approach to health.

One of the central pillars of hygienism is diet, which is no longer seen simply as a means of satisfying nutritional needs, but as an opportunity to actively support the body's self-healing process. By favouring a diet based on raw or lightly cooked and, above all, unprocessed foods, hygienism seeks to optimise digestion, strengthen the immune system and provide the body with the energy it needs to function at an optimal level. The aim is also to reduce toxaemia as much as possible, which is one of the biggest health problems today, and one that allopathic medicine does not address.

Rest and sleep also play a crucial role in the principles of hygienism. Sleep is seen as a time of essential and global regeneration, allowing the body to repair and revitalise its functions. Hygienism encourages regular and sufficient sleep habits to support physical and mental health.

Physical activity is another key element, not only for maintaining physical condition, but also for stimulating blood circulation, strengthening the cardiovascular system and promoting flexibility. However, hygienism stresses the importance of moderate exercise tailored to each individual, to avoid extremes that could lead to excessive stress on the body and the build-up of acids.

Stress management is an essential component of hygienism. Recognising the negative impact of chronic stress on health, this philosophy encourages regular relaxation, meditation and mindfulness practices to balance the nervous system and promote mental well-being.

Hygienism goes beyond the physical to encompass the emotional and social aspects of life. With its emphasis on healthy, fulfilling relationships, hygienism recognises the significant impact of positive social connections on mental and emotional well-being. Finally, an often-underestimated dimension is its commitment to ecology. By considering the impact of the environment on health, this philosophy encourages choices that respect the planet, promoting a balance between humanity and nature.

In short, hygienism offers a complete framework for living in harmony with the principles of health, well-being and the living world around us. By emphasising prevention, self-regeneration and conscious lifestyle choices, I propose a path towards sustainable vitality and holistic health that goes beyond the simple absence of disease to embrace a fulfilling life.

2. The laws of life and hygiene

2.1 *Enervation: impact on health and vitality*

Enervation, a key concept in the understanding of holistic health, refers to the depletion of an individual's vital energy. This condition can have profound consequences for physical, mental and emotional health, affecting the body's ability to maintain optimal internal balance. We will explore the links between enervation and various aspects of health, highlighting its impact on individual vitality.

Enervation occurs when the energy available for essential biological processes is insufficient. This energy deficiency can result from various factors such as chronic stress, an unbalanced lifestyle, or prolonged exposure to unfavourable conditions. It is crucial to understand that vital energy is the driving force behind detoxification, digestion, circulation and many other biological processes.

When enervation sets in, the body enters an energy-saving mode, prioritising detoxification functions to the detriment of other vital processes. This can lead to reduced intestinal transit, digestive problems, impaired blood circulation and a reduced ability to cope with stress. These physiological manifestations demonstrate how irritability can affect the whole body. In addition to the physical impacts, irritability has significant repercussions on mental health. Insufficient vital energy can lead to reduced sensory functions, persistent fatigue, restricted muscular capacity and reduced tolerance to stress. These psychological aspects are often overlooked, but they play an essential role in an individual's overall health.

When enervation persists, toxaemia, or the accumulation of toxic waste, increases excessively. The body then reacts with elimination attacks or acute illnesses, seeking to rapidly reduce toxaemia and promote a return to health. However, if enervation becomes chronic, vital energy is no longer distributed efficiently, leading to a cascade of symptoms and health problems.

Managing energy requires a holistic approach. Physical, mental and digestive rest are essential to restore vital energy: these are known as the three rests. Avoiding the absorption of toxic substances, whether through food or medication, is also crucial. Herbert M. Shelton stressed the importance of allowing the body to follow its own purification mechanisms rather than forcing it with artificial methods.

Biogony, or the life movements of the body, offers valuable insights into how the body responds to energy. Acute and chronic symptoms, inflammation and degenerative pathologies can all be interpreted through the prism of biogony. Understanding these movements allows practitioners to design tailored approaches to restoring health.

The impact of enervation goes beyond the physical body, also influencing the mental, emotional and energetic bodies. The specific needs of each body must be taken into account to maintain optimal health. Neglecting emotional, mental or energetic needs can lead to overall health problems, underlining the importance of a holistic approach to preventing enervation. In conclusion, enervation plays a central role in an individual's overall health. Understanding its mechanisms, its impact on the body and mind, and the ways in which it can be prevented and managed, is essential to promoting vitality and preventing the development of chronic illnesses. The holistic approach, integrating biogony and consideration of the subtle bodies, offers a comprehensive perspective to guide individuals towards an optimal state of health.

Dry fasting cures have been proposed as a way of stimulating the detoxification and self-healing process, allowing the body to free itself of accumulated toxins and restructure itself completely. During dry fasting, the body enters a state of ketosis, where it burns fat reserves to produce energy.

However, it is essential to recognise that dry fasting can initially cause a form of irritation. For the first few days, the body is adapting to the absence of food and water, which can lead to feelings of tiredness, headaches and other symptoms associated with detoxification. This initial phase can be interpreted as a period when vital energy is redirected towards cleansing and self-repair processes. In dry fasting, once this initial phase has been overcome, the body enters a regeneration phase. This is where potential health benefits such as reduced inflammation, regulation of metabolism and improved mental clarity are often observed, as well as a host of other benefits. Dry fasting can help reset the immune system and promote better management of vital energy in the long term.

During dry fasting cures, stress management becomes crucial. We recommend respecting the body's signals, getting enough rest and adopting the stress management practices we offer during our cures, which are constantly improving year after year. Holistic approaches such as meditation, yoga, kinesiology, gentle massage, ito thermie, breathing, personal development or therapeutic blanketing can be integrated to support energy balance during dry fasting.

It is important to note that the response to dry fasting can vary from person to person depending on various factors such as overall health, medical history and level of physical activity. Some individuals may feel more energetic, while others may experience a rapid improvement in vitality.

In conclusion, dry fasting cures can be associated with enervation, particularly during the initial adaptation phase. However, for many dry fasting practitioners, this period is seen as a necessary step towards regeneration and revitalisation. Careful management of vital energy during dry fasting, combined with a personalised approach, can help maximise the benefits while minimising the potential negative effects on enervation.

2.2 The importance of understanding toxaemia in order to heal and regain health

Toxaemia, or the accumulation of toxins in the body, can exceed an individual tolerance threshold, giving rise to various pathological symptoms. Rather than talking about the "four stages" of toxaemia, we can consider the "four levels of intoxication" to describe this progression.

1. **Initial Intoxication:** This first phase marks the beginning of a toxic build-up, where fatigue signals an alteration in overall health. This warning requires corrective measures such as rest, sufficient sleep, reduction of physical and

mental activities, and the adoption of a light diet or dry fasting to help detoxification.

2. **Acute reaction:** When the level of intoxication becomes intolerable, the body triggers a reaction in the form of an acute illness or crisis. This reaction is a defence mechanism designed to restore balance. Complete rest is then essential to facilitate the healing process and the return to an optimal state of health.

3. **Chronic phase:** If symptoms persist despite acute attacks, this indicates a chronic phase in which the body continually struggles to maintain the level of intoxication at a tolerable threshold. This stage reflects an inability to eliminate toxins completely, leading to a gradual deterioration in health.

4. **Advanced degeneration:** This last stage illustrates the negative evolution of chronic disorders towards serious and potentially fatal complications. It is characterised by persistent inflammation, ulceration, swelling and an increased risk of cancerous transformation, a sign of major systemic failure.

The naturopathic hygienic approach is considered to be a philosophy of life that promotes a set of conditions conducive to good health. It focuses on prevention by teaching the principles of vital hygiene, including nutrition, sleep, stress management and physical activity, to preserve vitality and avoid the onset of disease. This method emphasises that the state of health in which the level of toxaemia is a direct result of the lifestyle adopted illustrates the crucial importance of proactively and consciously taking care of one's well-being from the very first signs of imbalance.

2.3 *Solutions to reduce toxaemia*

Managing toxaemia, a condition resulting from the excessive accumulation of toxins in the body, requires a holistic approach that encompasses a healthy diet, stress and emotional management, sleep, physical exercise, and short and long dry fasts. Here's how to integrate these elements to improve your overall well-being.

Use of plants

Certain plants, such as dandelion, milk thistle, nettle and burdock, have detoxifying properties. They support the liver, kidneys and lymphatic system, making it easier to eliminate toxins.

Managing stress and emotions

Techniques such as meditation, yoga and deep breathing help to reduce stress, balance emotions and minimise the production of stress-related toxins.

Ideal, healthy diet

Eat a diet rich in fruit, vegetables, wholegrains and quality proteins. Avoid fermented foods and those rich in additives to maintain the body's pH balance and promote good digestion.

Restful sleep

A good night's sleep is crucial for the body's regeneration and the elimination of toxins. Adopt a regular bedtime routine and create an environment conducive to rest.

Physical exercise

Physical activity stimulates blood and lymph circulation, making it easier to eliminate toxins. Find an activity you enjoy and make it a regular part of your routine.

Hygiene techniques

Dry brushing the skin and detoxifying baths (with Epsom salt, for example) can stimulate circulation and help eliminate toxins through the skin.

Optimal mental health

Maintaining good mental health is essential. Consider therapies or support groups to manage stress and negative emotions.

Eliminating electromagnetic pollution

Reduce your exposure to electromagnetic fields by limiting the use of electronic devices and switching off Wi-Fi at night. Use wave protectors.

Social ties and inner calm

Cultivate positive relationships and take time for yourself. Practise gratitude and connect with nature to promote inner peace. Practise a 24-hour dry or water fast every week and an annual long dry fast. Seven days of dry fasting a year will allow your tissues and organs to be cleansed and renewed each year.

3. The experience of Alexis Carrel, French biologist

The experiment conducted by Alexis Carrel, the Nobel Prize-winning French biologist and surgeon, is often cited to illustrate the potential longevity of cells under optimal conditions. In the 1910s, Carrel began an experiment in which he kept chicken heart cells alive for an extended period using cell culture techniques and regularly replacing the nutrient medium in which the cells were grown.

Carrel's experiment demonstrated that as long as the cells were given an adequate nutrient environment and metabolic waste was regularly eliminated, they could survive and divide well beyond what was considered the normal lifespan for chicken cells. Some reports indicate that the cells were kept alive for more than 20 years, suggesting that in perfect conditions, with no toxins and adequate nutrients, human cells could potentially live well beyond 150 years.

This experiment has had a significant impact on science and medicine, highlighting the importance of the environment on health and cellular longevity. It has also fuelled discussions about the possibility of prolonging human life and methods of maintaining healthy tissues and organs. Living organisms are subject to a multitude of environmental, genetic and metabolic factors that influence their health and longevity.

Nevertheless, this experience illustrates the importance of effective toxin elimination, particularly through dry fasting, for maintaining good cellular health and, by extension, for the overall health of the body. It reinforces the idea that maintaining a clean environment, both internally and externally, while providing adequate nutrients, is essential for promoting longevity and preventing disease. Dry fasting is an ideal way to purify yourself and implement healthy habits in your physical and mental life.

Carrel's experiment offers a fascinating insight into the longevity of cells under optimal conditions, suggesting that a favourable environment can considerably prolong cell life. By keeping chicken heart cells alive for decades, well beyond their natural life expectancy, Carrel has highlighted the crucial importance of a suitable environment for cellular health and longevity. This work illustrates the potential for cells to live indefinitely in a toxin-free, nutrient-rich environment.

At the same time, dry fasting highlights a practical method by which individuals can positively influence their internal environment. By eliminating food and water intake for a period, dry fasting promotes detoxification and cellular regeneration. This practice creates internal conditions that are reminiscent, on a different scale, of the controlled environment that Alexis Carrel created for his chicken heart cells.

Dry fasting by promoting autophagy – the process by which cells break down and eliminate damaged components – can help to reduce accumulations of metabolic waste and improve cellular function.

Nevertheless, the analogy between the two approaches highlights a common fundamental principle: the need to adopt healthy lifestyle habits and maintain a pure internal environment to promote longevity and ageing well. Dry fasting offers an accessible route to improving overall health, echoing the lessons learned from Carrel's experience of the importance of a healthy environment for cellular longevity. By promoting a deep cleansing and revitalisation of the body, dry fasting can be seen as a concrete strategy for achieving optimal well-being and perhaps extending the length and quality of life.

4. Laws of Hippocrates – Fundamental principles of natural medicine

Remind your doctor when you see him or her.

1. **Vis medicatrix naturae – Nature's own** healing **power**
   Original: The body has the inherent ability to preserve health and restore it when it is lost.

   The body, by its very nature, has the intrinsic power to maintain health and to restore it in the event of imbalance. The vital forces at the heart of the body are essential allies in this process. The role of the doctor or therapist is to facilitate access to these forces by eliminating the obstacles that hinder them, rather than simply suppressing the symptoms, as contemporary medicine often does.

   Comment: Recognition of the regenerative power of nature inherent in our own bodies is a valuable guide to a holistic approach to healing. It reminds us that medicine should be a partnership with natural processes rather than an attempt to counteract them.

2. **Primum non nocere – First do no harm**
Original: The symptoms of an illness can be manifestations of a healing process. Simply suppressing them can do more harm than good.

Symptoms of illness, such as fever, can be signs of a healing process underway. So indiscriminate suppression of these symptoms can often result in more harm than benefit. Therapeutic interventions should therefore support the natural healing process rather than hinder it.

Comment: Prudence in medical intervention, avoiding harm to the natural healing processes, resonates as an essential ethical principle. It reminds us that the art of healing sometimes lies in the wisdom of not disturbing the intrinsic mechanisms of recovery. It is always useful to question the appropriateness of taking allopathic medicines.

3. **Tolle causam – Discovering and treating the cause**
Original: The doctor must look for the causes of the disease rather than trying to eliminate the symptoms.

Rather than simply treating the symptoms, the doctor must investigate and treat the underlying causes of the disease. Seeing illness as the ultimate result of a specific disorder, restoring the natural balance requires a targeted approach to the causes at the root of this disorder.

Comment: The approach of looking for underlying causes is a valuable reminder that medicine should not be limited to suppressing visible symptoms, but should instead focus on a deep understanding of the triggering factors in a holistic way.

4. **Deinde purgare – Detoxifying and purifying the body**
Comment: Detoxification, as advocated by Hippocrates, stresses the importance of freeing the body of accumulated impurities, allowing its natural healing mechanisms to function optimally.

5. **Docere** – Teaching
   Doctors must guide their patients along the road to recovery and help them to maintain their health in a natural way, while remaining the main players in their own recovery.
   The role of the doctor or therapist goes beyond treatment, and includes the duty to teach the patient how to take responsibility for his or her own health and healing process. This educational responsibility helps to empower the patient.
   Comment: The educational aspect of medicine is particularly important, as it empowers individuals to manage their own well-being, establishing a partnership between doctor and patient in the quest for optimal health.

5. Sporting activity

Physical activity and sport are key practices that should be incorporated into your life, both before and after dry fasting. Here are some key benefits.

1. **Helps maintain an optimal body weight**
   Regular physical activity can reduce the risk of becoming overweight or obese. Although exercise in itself does not necessarily guarantee spectacular weight loss, combined with a balanced, calorie-controlled diet, it can promote effective weight reduction. What's more, there is evidence to suggest that regular physical activity can help maintain a healthy body weight over the long term.

2. **It lowers blood pressure**
   High blood pressure, a risk factor for many diseases such as stroke and heart disease, can be reduced by regular physical activity. Regular exercise improves the strength

of the heart, reducing the effort needed to pump blood around the body. These benefits reduce the pressure exerted on the arteries, helping to maintain healthy blood pressure.

3. **It reduces the risk of heart disease**
   Regular exercise, particularly endurance activities such as brisk walking, running and cycling, has been shown to reduce the risk of developing heart disease. This benefit can be observed in individuals of all sizes, even those who are overweight or obese, underlining the importance of physical activity in preventing heart disease.

4. **It reduces the risk of type 2 diabetes**
   Exercise helps regulate blood sugar levels and increases insulin sensitivity, playing a crucial role in preventing type 2 diabetes. Conversely, physical inactivity is associated with an increased risk of developing the disease. People with diabetes can also benefit from regular exercise to control blood sugar levels.

5. **It reduces the risk of certain cancers**
   Evidence suggests that exercise at moderate or sustained intensity can help reduce the risk of colon, colorectal, lung and breast cancers. This underlines the importance of physical activity as a preventive measure against these complex diseases, which are influenced by a variety of factors.

6. **It increases muscle strength and function**
   Maintaining muscle mass is essential to prevent loss of mobility and reduce the risk of falls and age-related muscle diseases. Resistance training, including weightlifting and body weight exercises, can improve muscle strength and endurance, reducing the risk of muscular disorders such as sarcopenia.

7. **It improves bone health and density**
   Bodyweight exercise, such as running and dancing, as well as resistance training, have been shown to improve bone density in adolescents and maintain it in adults. This is particularly beneficial for older adults and post-menopausal women, helping to slow the natural loss of bone density associated with ageing.

8. **It promotes optimal mental health**
   Regular exercise has positive effects on mental health and psychological well-being by promoting the release of endorphins, relieving stress and encouraging healthy sleep patterns. In addition, there is evidence that exercise can play a role in the treatment of depression and other mental disorders.

9. **It reduces the risk of dementia**
   Regular exercise has been shown to protect against cognitive decline, probably through the release of neurotrophic factors. These proteins promote the growth and regeneration of neurons, helping to maintain normal cognitive function. This protection against cognitive decline may explain why older adults who remain physically active have a lower risk of developing cognitive disorders such as dementia or Alzheimer's disease.

10. **Improved quality of sleep**
    Regular exercise promotes deeper, more restful sleep. It helps to regulate sleep cycles, reducing insomnia problems and improving overall sleep quality.

11. **Boosting the immune system**
    Moderate physical activity strengthens the immune system by stimulating blood circulation, thereby promoting the

transport of immune cells throughout the body. This can help prevent infections and reduce the duration of illnesses.

12. **Increased energy and vitality**
    Regular exercise improves blood circulation, which increases the supply of oxygen and nutrients to the cells. This leads to a general increase in energy and vitality, helping to combat fatigue and improve day-to-day productivity.

13. **Reduced stress and anxiety**
    Physical activity releases endorphins, the feel-good neurotransmitters that reduce stress and anxiety. Regular exercise sessions can serve to free the mind by encouraging a positive state of mind.

14. **Improving flexibility and mobility**
    Exercises that focus on flexibility, such as yoga and stretching, help to maintain an optimal range of movement. This is particularly important for preventing injury and maintaining mobility over time.

15. **Strengthening the cardiorespiratory system**
    Cardiovascular exercise improves the efficiency of the cardiorespiratory system, increasing lung capacity and strengthening the heart. This leads to better endurance and increased resistance to physical activity.

16. **Promoting healthy digestion**
    Regular physical activity can help regulate intestinal transit, promoting healthy digestion. This can help prevent gastrointestinal problems such as constipation.

17. **Strengthening the musculoskeletal system**
    In addition to the effect on muscle mass, exercise helps to strengthen joints, ligaments and bones, reducing the risk of injury and joint diseases such as arthritis.

18. **Improving posture and balance**
    Activities such as muscle strengthening and coordination help to improve posture and balance. This can help prevent back pain and falls, especially among the elderly.

19. **Reduction in insulin**
    Regular exercise improves insulin sensitivity. When you exercise, your muscles need more glucose to function. To allow glucose to enter the cells, the body increases insulin sensitivity. This means that less insulin is needed to regulate blood sugar levels. In the long term, this can help to reduce circulating insulin levels.

20. **Improved glucose management**
    Physical activity helps to regulate blood glucose levels. During and after exercise, the muscles use glucose as a source of energy, helping to lower blood sugar levels. This regulation of glucose can have positive effects on insulin secretion.

21. **Reduction in glycated haemoglobin (HbA1c)**
    HbA1c is a measure of average blood glucose levels over a period of two to three months. Regular exercise, by improving insulin sensitivity and regulating blood sugar levels, can help maintain lower HbA1c levels. This is particularly important for people with type 2 diabetes or pre-diabetes, as high HbA1c levels are associated with an increased risk of diabetes-related complications.

The Benefits and Advantages of Dry Fasting

Dry fasting offers a multitude of benefits for physical, mental, and emotional health, far surpassing the advantages of water fasting. Here is an exhaustive and enhanced list of its benefits:

- **Effective Stimulation of Healing and Recovery Processes**: Dry fasting boosts the body's resistance by strengthening the immune system, accelerating healing, and speeding up the recovery from illnesses.
- **Protection Against Psycho-Emotional Factors**: It helps combat burnout, depression, and other psycho-emotional disorders, bringing mental clarity and emotional well-being.
- **Treatment of Chronic Conditions and Diseases**: Dry fasting is effective in treating various painful conditions and chronic diseases at different stages of development. Although a single cure may sometimes be insufficient, it often lays the foundation for deeper healing.
- **Regeneration and Rejuvenation of Organs and Tissues**: It enhances and restores the processes of regeneration and repair, leading to visible rejuvenation of the skin and body tissues.
- **Prevention of Metabolic Disorders**: Dry fasting acts as a general preventive measure against metabolic disorders, helping to maintain a balanced metabolism.
- **Overall Strengthening and Rejuvenation**: It strengthens and rejuvenates the body, acting as a powerful and natural anti-aging remedy without equal.

- **Weight Loss and Metabolism Restoration**: Dry fasting helps shed excess weight by restoring metabolism and promoting sustainable weight loss.
- **Combating Addictions**: It is effective in fighting unhealthy habits and addictions, whether to food, alcohol, cigarettes, or sugary products.
- **A New Lease on Life**: Dry fasting leads to significant and conscious life changes, helping individuals rediscover their full vital and mental potential.
- **Improvement of the Musculoskeletal System**: It improves the functioning of the musculoskeletal system, helping to combat osteochondrosis, osteoporosis, arthritis, and aiding in rehabilitation after severe injuries.
- **Metabolism Regulation and Cellular Reset**: Dry fasting regulates the entire metabolism, promoting a cellular reset and facilitating weight gain or loss as needed.
- **Overall Detoxification**: It detoxifies the body, providing both physical and mental relief, and promotes a slimmer figure with rapid weight loss.
- **Elimination of Heavy Metals and Toxins**: Dry fasting detoxifies heavy metals, pollutants, and physical and psychic toxins, helping to deeply cleanse the body.
- **Ideal for Electrosensitive Individuals**: It helps restore cells to their original state, proving particularly beneficial after exposure to high levels of radioactivity, as demonstrated by post-Chernobyl experience.
- **Effective Against Infections**: Dry fasting is effective against all types of infections, whether viral, parasitic, or bacterial, and is particularly useful in cases of chronic Lyme disease.
- **Sports Preparation**: It deeply cleanses the body and improves mitochondria, potentially prolonging the careers of athletes nearing the end of their careers.

- **DNA and Mitochondrial Renewal**: Dry fasting works at the level of DNA and mitochondria, creating a complete renewal of the organism.
- **Natural Anti-Inflammatory Effect**: It relieves chronic pain due to its powerful natural anti-inflammatory effect.
- **Return to Self and Mental Clarity**: Dry fasting helps to clarify thoughts, fosters self-awareness, and aids in better self-understanding.
- **Improvement of Lifestyle Habits**: It encourages better lifestyle habits and helps establish new healthy dietary structures.
- **Annual Prevention**: An annual course of dry fasting can maintain excellent physical and mental health.
- **General Anti-Aging Effect**: By multiplying the cures, dry fasting can act as a powerful anti-aging agent, slowing the effects of aging.
- **Rehabilitation of Athletes**: It is effective for athletes suffering from chronic pain or having medical diagnoses that limit their careers, potentially getting them back on their feet even at an advanced age.

In conclusion, dry fasting offers a holistic and powerful approach to improving physical, mental, and emotional health, far surpassing the benefits of water fasting. Whether for healing diseases, detoxification, weight loss, or rejuvenation, dry fasting stands out as an incomparable therapeutic method among all existing natural therapies. It remains a unique system of self-repair for the body, unknown to most people.

CHAPTER 2

What is dry fasting?

Dry fasting, also known as waterless fasting, is a practice in which a person abstains from all solid and liquid foods for a set period of time. Unlike intermittent fasting, which generally allows the consumption of water, dry fasting excludes all water intake, and this is its strength compared with other types of fasting.

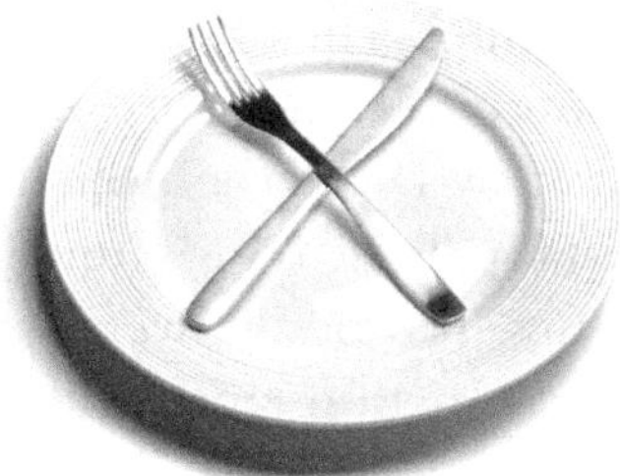

During dry fasting, the body uses its internal reserves to obtain the necessary energy and produce water. This includes breaking down stored fat and mobilising glycogen. The absence of external input forces the metabolism to adapt, resulting in hormonal and metabolic changes. This practice has powerful health benefits and is currently the most successful self-healing method available in therapeutic terms. It reduces inflammation, treats infections, stimulates autophagy and renovates organs much more rapidly than water fasting.

1. Dry fasting and general information

Fasting, defined as the total abstention from solid or liquid foods other than pure water, or even the total abstention from all foods including pure water, over periods of varying length, offers a salutary approach to health. It constitutes a restriction, or even a momentary elimination, of solid food, recommended to promote better health and offer a first-level healing method. Dry fasting is particularly indicated in various contexts, such as obesity, cardiovascular disease, detoxification and kidney and intestinal disorders.

Introducing periods of fasting into the year, combined with a reduction in the amount of food eaten, initiates a detoxification of the body, offering notable results such as weight loss, improved blood quality, rejuvenated skin, consolidation of old fractures, improved physical and intellectual fitness, and the confidence to live well. It also boosts resistance to disease. The hygienic fasting model advocated by Dr Herbert Shelton emphasises the importance of total rest for all the body's functions during fasting.

In a state of fasting, the body saves the energy generally allocated to muscular function and makes it available for the function of eliminating toxins. Physical activity is not recommended during a state of acidosis resulting from stress and diet.

During dry fasting, the body works in slow motion. The duration of dry fasting depends on the patient's vitality, age, reserves and the illness to be treated. It is crucial to avoid dry fasting in cases of excessive fatigue, as elimination and renewal require energy, and fasting can become counterproductive.

Therapeutic dry fasting resolves many common health problems, promoting tissue regeneration and improving physiological functions. It is best to start with short dry fasts before embarking on a long dry fast.

Dry fasting is only a means to an end: it prepares the body for a correct and healthy lifestyle. The benefits of dry fasting depend on the post-fasting lifestyle, with a healthy diet, appropriate physical exercise, fresh air, mental and physical rest, and the elimination of devitalising habits. Dry fasting can prevent ageing, rejuvenating the body and contributing to a more youthful appearance.

In conclusion, dry fasting, as a process of cleansing and physiological rest, offers a holistic approach to preserving and restoring health. Its benefits extend beyond simple abstention from food, having a positive impact on intellectual and emotional qualities. The post-fasting balance, characterised by a healthy lifestyle and healthy hygiene, determines the duration of the beneficial results, underlining the importance of maintaining health-promoting lifestyle habits. The post-dry fasting state is crucial. Once dry fasting is over, it is essential to make micro-changes and avoid returning to an unbalanced diet and a sedentary lifestyle.

2. Dry fasting, a little history

Present throughout the history of religions, it is often associated with ascetic, spiritual and purifying practices. Although the specific details vary, dry fasting has been adopted by some followers of different religious traditions in search of physical and spiritual purification.

In the context of Christianity, the Gospels mention that Jesus Christ fasted for 40 days in the desert. This period of fasting is often interpreted as a test of physical and spiritual endurance, demonstrating inner strength in the face of temptation. Although the biblical texts do not specify whether Jesus abstained completely from water during this period, his fast is generally considered to be an example of spiritual discipline.

In Judaism, fasting is also practised on various occasions, with Yom Kippur (the Day of Atonement) representing one of the most important fasts. During this day, the faithful abstain from food and drink, emphasising the quest for purification and repentance.

In Islam, fasting is a well-known practice during the month of Ramadan. Muslims observe a daily fast, abstaining from food and drink from sunrise to sunset. Although this fast mainly involves abstaining from food and drink, it can also be seen as a form of dry fasting during the daytime hours. There are numerous scientific studies on the benefits of short dry fasts, which you can find on pub med.

Buddhism, with its various schools and traditions, also has stories of practitioners who observed periods of strict fasting in order to reach a higher state of consciousness and understanding. In his spiritual quest, Siddhartha Gautama followed severe asceticism, including periods of fasting, before his enlightenment.

The stories of religious figures who practised dry fasting are not limited to these examples. Sages, mystics and hermits from various traditions have also explored this practice as a way of transcending bodily needs and deepening their spiritual connection.

Vision seeking is a shamanic practice that varies from culture to culture, but is often used to obtain visions, spiritual insights or answers to important questions. Vision quests can take many forms, but generally involve voluntary isolation in the wilderness, often combined with periods of fasting, meditation, chanting, dancing or other ritual practices.

Fasting, and dry fasting in particular, can be incorporated into a vision quest for a number of reasons. Some shamans believe that fasting can purify the body and mind, making them more receptive to spiritual energies or visions. In addition, fasting can be seen as a way of demonstrating the spiritual seeker's determination and commitment to the vision quest.

It is important to note that practices vary considerably according to the cultures and shamanic traditions of certain countries and regions. Ultimately, the vision quest in shamanism is often aimed at enabling the practitioner to enter into contact with the spiritual world, to receive guidance, visions or answers to questions that are important for their personal life or for their community. Dry fasting is a well-known response to the need for deep introspection and open states of consciousness.

3. The history of modern dry fasting with Russia.

In Russia, Professor Viktor Vasilevic Pašutin and his colleagues made the greatest scientific contribution to the study of experimental dry fasting at the end of the 19th century. In turn, Pašutin, a pupil of Professor S.P. Botkin, the most famous physician of the time who worked at the Czarist Russian Military Medical Academy, spent a long time experimenting with dry fasting on various animals and formulating the essence of its physiological mechanisms. Pašutin soon noticed for the first time that during the first period of fasting there is a rapid loss of weight, but that this loss diminishes after a few days. At the time, the mechanisms that preserve energy and reduce weight loss were not yet clear. But studies were already showing that the body's protein consumption during this period is kept to a minimum, and cells, including those in the nervous tissue and endocrine system, do not suffer.

If the limits of physiological fasting in animals are exceeded, a third phase occurs, during which there is a sharp reduction in body weight associated with the exhaustion of compensatory mechanisms and degeneration of cardiac activity. The distinction between these three phases characteristic of absolute fasting in mammals makes Pašutin the precursor of the theory of dry fasting or endogenous nutrition. His experiments have lost none of their importance to this day. In subsequent experiments carried out on different living beings, it was shown that the first two physiological stages of fasting in different living beings occur at different times. Thanks to these periods of fasting, the lifespan is extended compared with that of organisms that eat regularly. For example, fasting can extend the lifespan of worms by 19 times, of mice by four times and of mammals by 1.5 to two times.

A hundred years ago, Pašutin also noted that pathologically altered tissues are consumed during fasting. It is precisely the elimination of old, diseased, dead, weak and decaying tissue from the body that guarantees a powerful therapeutic effect. During this process, the healthy tissues not only do not suffer, but also benefit, as they are renewed. Hence the rejuvenating effect that everyone reports, making dry fasting one of the new treatment methods of our time. A de facto method born at the dawn of humanity and used by all representatives of the animal kingdom at the beginning of the development of the animal life forms that exist today. A common feature of all types of fasting is the use of *"tissue stocks"* or, to use F. Benedict's definition, the transition to an endogenous diet, which uses the energetic and plastic substances released during the slow atrophy of a certain part of the body's tissues and structures. The intensity of the atrophic changes (simple atrophy) in the various organs and tissues is generally proportional to the duration of the fast.

It has been established that during fasting there is a change in the orientation of endogenous nutrition between organs. The main proof of this principle is the fact that when animals die of starvation, there is an exceptionally different weight loss in the various organs and tissues. The greatest losses occur in adipose tissue (97% of initial weight), liver and spleen (53-60%), skeletal muscle (30%), blood (26%), kidney (25%), skin (20%), intestine (18%), bone (13%), nervous system (3.9%), heart (3.6%), while brain tissue loses virtually no weight. An exceptionally important constant has thus been discovered: the expenditure of the internal reserves of the various organs and tissues is by no means uniform. The more important an organ or tissue is for vital functions, the less weight it loses, and vice versa, i.e. organs and tissues of vital importance continue to exist indefinitely at the expense of secondary tissues and organs.

The in-depth restructuring of metabolic processes during fasting aims to optimise the use of reserve substances and to limit as far as possible the needs of organs and tissues which are less important for the preservation of life. When substances are redistributed from less important organs to more vital organs, a reduction in body weight loss has been observed. Fed after repeated fasting, the animals reached a higher body weight, and their tissues became more compact than before. When the animals were fed after several periods of fasting, a marked increase in metabolic processes was also noted. Pašutin observed that: *"the tissues of the nervous centres and sense organs use reserves from other parts of the body in abundance, maintaining their weight status quo until the last moments of fasting. The significance of this state of neural resistance is understandable. The nervous system is predisposed to the development of special forces, with which it manages the activity of almost every part of the body. For this reason, it is natural that, given this important function, it should not have purely alimentary tasks such as supplying different substances with blood".* Thus, Pašutin's findings on dry fasting focused mainly on the impact of food deprivation on the body's metabolic processes and physiology. Pašutin, renowned for his significant contributions to pathophysiology, studied how fasting affects the body's reserves and the redistribution of substances in the organs.

Here are a few key points from his observations and discoveries:

1. **Restructuring of metabolic processes:** Pašutin has noted that fasting leads to a profound restructuring of metabolic processes. The body uses its reserves optimally, reducing the needs of organs and tissues that are less vital for the preservation of life. During the redistribution of substances from less important organs to vital organs, a reduction in body weight loss is observed.

2. **Use of body reserves:** Pašutin observed that the tissues of the nerve centres and sense organs use reserves from other parts of the body, maintaining their weight until the last moments of fasting. This indicates neural resistance and the priority of the nervous system in managing bodily resources during fasting.

3. **Capacity of the body to use up reserves:** The work of Pašutin and other physiologists has shown that the body can use up 40-45% of its weight before reaching a state of total decomposition. Dry fasting with a loss of body weight of up to 20-25% is considered to pose no pathological risk to health. For example, an individual weighing 80 kg at the start could easily drop to 60 kg, without risk.

4. **Distinction between dosed and pathological fasting: Pašutin** drew a distinction between dosed fasting, where no pathological changes occur, and pathological fasting, which can lead to dystrophy and death. Metered fasting is used in a controlled setting to take advantage of the positive effects of food deprivation without causing damage.

5. **Impact on homeostasis:** The maintenance of homeostasis during fasting is generally summarised as the maintenance of the body's "firm constants", despite changes in the "labile constants". These discoveries laid the foundations for the modern understanding of fasting and its effects on the human body. They also inspired subsequent practices and research into the health benefits of fasting.

- **Porfirij Ivanov 1898- 1983**

In Soviet times, academician Pašutin's interest in the mechanisms of fasting was put into practice by Porfirij Ivanov, founder of a unique healing system that also included dry fasting. Born at the end of the 19th century in Ukraine into a family of miners, he went to work after only four parish classes. Until the age of 36 he lived an ordinary life, but always thought about how he could help people to live a better life, not to fall ill and not to die young. In 1934, he had a recurring dream that made him realise that man must not fight against the negative factors of nature, but must learn to exploit them for his own benefit. He began to experiment with different procedures for tempering the body:

he went out without a helmet, walked barefoot all year round, without a coat in winter, and even poured cold water over his body during that season.

He developed phenomenal powers of resistance: he could stop eating and drinking for a fortnight, stay two-three hours in water in the sea in winter. He even spent hours on the steppe in the middle of a snowstorm, covered only in his underwear. He's run hundreds of kilometres on dirt tracks in winter, stripped naked. He travelled for hours on locomotives. We know that during the Nazi occupation, he was buried half-naked in the snow and was transported by motorbike, but he didn't even catch a cold. As well as developing iron health, his remarkable bioenergetic and extrasensory abilities helped him to cure complex illnesses: a case of chronic leg paralysis, psoriasis, ulcers, cases of tuberculosis, stomach cancer and much more.

He lived through a period that did not allow his extraordinary abilities to manifest themselves. These were the years of the revolution, the terror of the political police, the Second World War and the last years of the totalitarian regime of the Communist Party. He was arrested several times and spent 12 years in prison in psychiatric hospitals, but nothing could destroy him. He tried to divulge his ideas in the press, but it was almost impossible in those years of rigorous administrative management. He had hundreds of followers to whom he passed on his doctrine (Detka).

- **Dr Jurij Nikolaev 1920-1998**

An important role in the spread of therapeutic fasting, both wet and dry, was played by the famous psychiatrist Jurij Nikolaev, who in 1960 devoted his doctoral thesis to the physiological basis of the application of fasting in the treatment of schizophrenia. Fascinated by Eastern culture and yogic lifestyles, and the author of numerous scientific articles on the beneficial effects of decongestant therapy, Nikolaev began to successfully introduce therapeutic fasting into psychiatric practice. He worked at the Ministry of the USSR Institute of Health and continued to disseminate his research at the Chair of Psychiatry at the Rostov and then Moscow Medical Institutes, creating around him a veritable school of highly qualified psychiatrists and therapists. The latter succeeded in opening specialised fasting departments in many urban and regional hospitals.

In 1990, his book "Golodanie radi zdorov'ja" (Fasting for health) was published in Rostov, written with other co-authors. Nikolaev occupies a special place in the history of Russian medicine. He succeeded in changing the approach to fasting by demonstrating its therapeutic properties in psychiatric illnesses. His contribution has been recognised by specialists in Japan and Germany. In India, where Nikolaev was a frequent guest, he was made an honorary member of the Yoga Institute. In the United States, he was appointed an ordinary member of the Academy of Orthomolecular (Rehabilitation).

- **Prof. Ščennikov, 1929-2019**

The greatest contribution to the development of the therapeutic dry fasting method was made by L.A. Ščennikov. His method of therapeutic abstinence (patent no. 2028160: "Method of rehabilitation of the organism"), validated in 1992, is well known in many Russian cities and abroad. Ščennikov is a biologist and expert in non-traditional medicine, naturopath and healer.

For more than 40 years, he has been demonstrating the benefits of therapeutic abstinence at the cellular level of the body, confirmed by the results of experiments carried out by medical research institutes and by the discoveries of followers of this technique. These results are also confirmed by people who have embarked on a path of self-healing and self-discovery, which has enabled them to acquire solid health and a new quality of perception of life. Ščennikov carried out a 21-day dry fast without food or water at his home in the Caucasus. He has accompanied thousands of fasters in this process of therapeutic fasting and has filed the only patent recognised by his country as a method of health rehabilitation, which you can find later in this book.

4. Fasting has always been practised

Today, therapeutic dry fasting is considered to be one of the most effective healing methods in the world, although few people have really understood its power. Yet this approach is "as old as the hills". It was born at the dawn of humanity. We can say with certainty that since the beginning of the evolution of the animal life forms that exist today, dry fasting has been frequently used by all their representatives.

What does an injured animal do in the wild? It rests and leaves its body to recover. There are no water fountains, coffee machines or food nearby. Energy is recovered through physical and digestive rest. This process is incorporated into the genetic code of animals and humans.

As humanity progressed, this archaic method was largely forgotten, and it is only in recent decades, thanks to the growing popularity of hygienism and water fasting, that interest in this ancient practice has returned.

When the body falls ill, it begins to mobilise all its forces to protect itself and starts to use up its reserves, if any. Consequently, in order to save energy for processing external food and water, the body triggers a rescue programme, which involves an automatic "refusal" to consume anything. Similar situations also occur in response to unfavourable environmental conditions, to protect themselves from extreme cold (winter hibernation) or extreme heat. Animals do not eat or drink for long periods and enter a state of inactivity and metabolic depression characterised by low body temperature, slow respiration and heart rate, and a low metabolic rate. The function of hibernation-estivation is to conserve energy when food is unavailable in sufficient quantities.

- **Key mechanisms of dry fasting and physiology**

The physiology of dry fasting is a complex process involving several body systems. One of the most interesting aspects of dry fasting is the body's ability to synthesise water.

- **Endogenous water metabolism**

During a dry fast, the body begins to produce endogenous water. This water is generated by burning fat reserves stored in the body. When these fats, composed of carbon, hydrogen and oxygen, are metabolised for energy, they break down into carbon dioxide (exhaled through the lungs) and water. The hydrogen in fat combines with the oxygen we breathe in to form water, a process known as fat oxidation.

- **Water conservation and body adaptation**

In the absence of water intake, the body puts mechanisms in place to conserve water. This includes reducing urine production and reducing water loss by other means, such as sweating and breathing. The kidneys thus play a crucial role in adjusting the concentration and volume of urine. During a dry fast, the body switches from a state in which it derives most of its energy from carbohydrates to a state in which it uses stored fats as its main source of energy. This process is called ketosis. The ketone bodies produced during ketosis can provide energy for the brain and other organs.

- **Weight loss**

The rapid weight loss observed during dry fasting is due in part to the loss of water and fat. As the body uses fat reserves for energy, the amount of water retained in these tissues is also released and used.

- **Cleansing and detoxification**

Dry fasting is also considered to be a novel and ultra-powerful cleansing process, in which the body eliminates accumulated toxins. The absence of new food intake allows the digestive system to rest and the detoxification organs, such as the liver and kidneys, to work more efficiently.

- **Immune and anti-inflammatory responses**

Dry fasting can influence the body's immune and anti-inflammatory responses. The absence of food can reduce inflammation and modulate the immune system, which is potentially beneficial for certain autoimmune and inflammatory conditions. Dry fasting can reduce levels of pro-inflammatory cytokines in the body. This reduction in systemic inflammation is beneficial for the immune system, as chronic inflammation can weaken the immune response and is associated with various chronic diseases.

Dry fasting also allows the following mechanisms:

1. **Increased autophagy:** Autophagy is a cellular cleansing process in which cells break down and recycle damaged or dysfunctional components. Dry fasting stimulates autophagy three to five times more than water fasting, which can help eliminate intracellular pathogens and maintain cellular homeostasis, thereby boosting immune health.

2. **Regeneration of immune cells:** Studies on animal models and a few human studies suggest that fasting can stimulate the regeneration of new immune cells. This is particularly apparent after prolonged periods of fasting, when the body breaks down and recycles ageing immune cells and replaces them with new ones.

3. **Modulation of the intestinal microbiota:** Fasting can influence the composition of the intestinal microbiota, which plays a crucial role in regulating the immune response. Changes in the microbiota can have an impact on immunity by altering the production of metabolites and signalling molecules that affect the immune system.

4. **Reduced oxidative stress:** Fasting can reduce oxidative stress by reducing the production of free radicals and increasing the body's antioxidant mechanisms. A reduction in oxidative stress can have a positive effect on the immune system by protecting immune cells from damage.

5. **Changes in hormone levels:** Fasting influences several hormones involved in regulating the immune response, such as insulin, glucagon and corticosteroids. These hormonal changes can have an impact on the activity of the immune system.

5. Is fasting with Buchinger-type juices and broths, tea and lemon really fasting?

No, it's a diet with more or fewer calories. The body works by an all-or-nothing mechanism. Either we fast with water or we fast dry. If we take a drink, juice or tea and add it to the water, the body perceives it as food and the autolysis and autophagy phases will be slowed down and all the precious benefits of fasting will be slowed down, with possible cravings for food which may make fasting more complicated, because digestive secretions are activated with a lesser therapeutic effect and insulin will also rise and all the fasting mechanisms will be slowed down. Cell membranes function only with water, or without water by creating endogenous water. Adding a liquid or juice is tantamount to a diet, no more and no less.

In my experience, juice and broth-based diets only bring digestive improvement and a slight detox. Even long diets of four weeks will have a soothing effect but will not resolve chronic pathological conditions. This type of fast cannot resolve the underlying causes of imbalance. The one-week diets proposed everywhere are wellness diets, useful for preparing for real fasting, but they do not constitute a complete and global path to healing.

6. What are the advantages of dry fasting over wet fasting?

During a dry fast, the body is subjected to much harsher conditions than during a water fast. The Law of Hormesis shows us that the harder the dry fast, the greater the restorative response. The body is forced to restructure itself in order to produce not only nutrients, but also water. Cell division in the body's tissues takes place more rapidly and in a shorter space of time. The phases of therapeutic fasting, in the case of dry fasting, are identical to those of water fasting, but the timescales are considerably reduced: the excitation phase lasts less than a day, the phase of increasing ketosis lasts from one to three days, and the ketotic crisis appears on the third day of dry fasting. The second acidotic crisis, the most curative, occurs between days nine and 11. The earlier it occurs, the faster it passes, leaving more time for the body to renew and heal itself.

During a water fast, exogenous water (from outside) enters the body, and water is the main purifying agent. According to the law of biological efficiency, a cell in this case expends the minimum amount of energy: all the toxins, poisons and waste are dissolved, and, to put it graphically, there is a phenomenon of washing the toxins from the cells and the intercellular space. However, during a dry fast, the incineration of toxins takes place in their own oven, as it were. This means that each cell, in the absence of water, triggers an internal fusion reaction and is transformed into a mini-reactor. Water is extremely necessary and cells are deprived of it, which is particularly problematic for diseased and altered cells. In these extreme circumstances, the strongest and healthiest cells survive, and to survive in this situation they have to intensify the production of their own high-quality endogenous water. This endogenous water is probably of much higher quality than the exogenous water, again according to the law of biological efficiency. A cell consumes a lot of energy, so the resulting product must match the effort invested in quality. We are not dealing here with the human mind, which can make mistakes, but with a natural process that oversees every stage of development and aims to ensure the continuation of life.

Many patients report that dry fasting is better tolerated than water fasting because there is no sensation of hunger, and this is not surprising. In fact, exogenous water and the body's own water are very different. When the body receives water from outside, it has to rework the molecules, erase the unnecessary information, structure them and transform them into 'proprietary' molecules with the body's own properties. To do this, as with digesting food, the body is obliged to expend a certain amount of energy and time. With dry fasting, all these processes do not occur and in this sense it is a more complete practice because it offers total rest to the body. If no food or heavy ("dead") water enters the body, the blood receives no harmful substances and has the chance to be constantly cleansed by the body. The blood composition is constantly purified through the filtration systems and becomes perfectly pure. During dry fasting, the blood eliminates all superfluous substances and the blood plasma becomes as transparent as glass, everything is reharmonised, including the coagulation factors. Dry fasting purifies the blood more thoroughly than a blood purification treatment, haemodialysis or haemabsorption.

The anti-inflammatory effect of dry fasting is much more powerful than the effect obtained with wet fasting. This is because inflammation cannot exist without water. Inflamed areas swell. Micro-organisms, such as microbes and viruses, can only multiply in a sufficiently watery environment. It follows that a lack of water is extremely counterproductive for the inflammatory process. With dry fasting, the lack of external water means that pathogenic micro-organisms immediately find an unfavourable environment. Thanks to the dehydration caused by dry fasting, the body's cells and the pathogenic micro-organisms enter into a very severe competition for water. The body's cells can easily seize water from micro-organisms and much more besides. In dry fasting mode, the body not only synthesises endogenous water, but can also acquire it from the air, by absorption through the skin. This is because during dry fasting, the skin stops secreting water and switches to absorption mode. Healthy, strong cells receive an extra dose of energy and water, while sick cells, viruses, bacteria and parasites cannot. Microbes, viruses, worms and parasites die instantly without water, which is why dry fasting can also be used as an emergency treatment for infections. It remains a subject to be explored by scientists who are genuinely looking out for the good of humankind and not to make big pharma fat.

During dry fasting, these treatments are not necessary because the body triggers its own unique mechanisms which neutralise poisons and toxins. This does not happen in any other form of fasting. During dry fasting, the toxins burn in their own oven: each cell, in the absence of water, triggers an internal thermal reaction. The result is a kind of extreme and immediate destruction, within the cells themselves, of all waste, superfluous and pathological elements. Each cell is temporarily transformed into a mini-reactor and the body's internal temperature rises. This change in temperature may not be detected by a thermometer, but during dry fasting, patients feel it as internal heat, 'fire' or shivering. Temperature is an integral part of a series of defensive reactions. From experience, we know that fever eliminates all toxins; poisons and even tumour cells completely suspend their activity. This process accelerates healing. By reacting with fever, the body slows down the growth of micro-organisms.

7. What is the difference between pranism and dry fasting?

Pranism and dry fasting are two practices that aim to modify the traditional approach to food and nutrition, but they do so in very different ways and with distinct objectives. Pranism is based on the belief that it is possible for an individual to live without food or water, feeding solely on subtle energies, often called 'prana' in Hindu traditions or 'chi' in Chinese traditions. Practitioners of pranism seek to transcend traditional physical needs to achieve a state of non-dependence on food. This practice is often associated with profound spiritual searches and aims to bring about a radical transformation of the human being. It is not generally seen as a therapeutic method, but rather as a long-term life path. However, it is important to note that this practice is extremely controversial and considered by the medical community to be potentially dangerous, as the human body requires nutritional inputs to function properly over a lifetime. Only a few scholars in India seem capable of such feats. In the West, some people claim to be 'pranic', but you really need to be able to follow these people in detail, as some take juices or foods, so be wary of impostors.

Dry fasting, on the other hand, consists of abstaining from all food and liquids, including water, for a limited period never exceeding 11 days. This practice is often used for reasons of health, purification or therapy, and above all for health prevention. Advocates of dry fasting argue that this method allows the body to cleanse and regenerate itself, by drawing on its internal reserves and eliminating toxins. Unlike pranism, dry fasting is practised over short periods, generally from a few days to a few weeks, and is followed by a period of controlled resumption of eating to allow the body to readapt to food. Fans of dry fasting often report a boost in energy and increased well-being after the fasting period, although these claims vary greatly from person to person.

Interestingly, some people may experience a period of devitalisation after prolonged pranism. This could be because, unlike dry fasting where the body adapts temporarily to the absence of food and water, pranism aims for a permanent cessation of food over the long term, which can lead to severe nutritional deficiencies and a deterioration in health.

It is crucial to stress that these practices require a thorough understanding of their potential impact on health and should be approached with caution. The supervision of a health professional is strongly recommended, especially for people wishing to experiment with dry fasting. As for pranism, given the significant health risks involved in becoming pranic and living for years without eating, it is important to carefully consider the motivations and possible consequences before embarking on such a practice.

Beware of pseudo dry fasting experts on the internet and on fasting websites. Implementing and monitoring dry fasting requires rigour and practical expertise. The importance of qualified expertise in dry fasting cannot be underestimated. Only therapists who have themselves practised dry fasting, who actively accompany dry fasting patients and who have solid experience in counselling, are truly credible in this field. These professionals not only have an intimate understanding of the challenges and benefits of dry fasting, they also have the experience to identify and manage the risks. Some of them have even written books or articles on fasting, or published YouTube videos in which they explain how to fast, without having fasted for more than 24 hours themselves, let alone having followed fasters on a cure. Always check that the person accompanying you ticks all the boxes in terms of experience, otherwise what the person says will have little credibility. It is risky and misleading to observe that someone has successfully fasted dry for a long period of time with certain benefits, and to naively believe that it is possible to match or replicate exactly their experience, the same benefits and the duration of their fast. Each individual is unique, and reactions to dry fasting can vary considerably.

Dry fasting can offer many health benefits, including detoxification and cellular and complete regeneration of the body. However, it also presents risks, as you must not exceed your own capacity to adapt. This requires careful monitoring and management. Experienced therapists are able to assess each individual, personalise dry fasting programmes and provide appropriate follow-up, taking into account physical, emotional and psychological aspects. Before embarking on such a programme, it is essential to consult an experienced professional to ensure that the practice is suitable and safe.

The impact of fat breakdown during dry fasting to create endogenous water

During this period of fasting, the body has to adapt to meet its energy and water requirements without any external input.

Contrary to what you might think, dehydration is often avoided thanks to internal mechanisms for regulating and redistributing water, because let's not forget that the human body is 60-70% water.

During a dry fast, the body begins to use fat reserves as its main source of energy. This process is called lipolysis, in which the triglycerides stored in the fat cells are broken down into fatty acids and glycerol. The fatty acids released during lipolysis undergo oxidation to produce energy. A by-product of this oxidation is metabolic water. The body therefore generates internal water during the breakdown of fat.

It is estimated that the complete oxidation of 100 grams of fat can produce around 107 to 110 millilitres of metabolic water. This can help maintain water balance in the body during dry fasting.

This process, called beta-oxidation, takes place in the mitochondria. Each beta-oxidation cycle shortens the fatty acid by two carbon atoms, producing acetyl-CoA, NADH and FADH2. Acetyl-CoA enters the Krebs cycle, where it is transformed to produce more NADH and FADH2. These reduced coenzymes transport electrons to the electron transport chain, generating ATP and water as a by-product. The simplified reaction for the formation of water is :

This metabolic water contributes significantly to maintaining body hydration during dry fasting, as the body adapts by reducing water loss through urine and perspiration. The kidneys become more efficient at conserving water and maintaining homeostasis while performing a gentle detoxification. The body uses water conservation mechanisms, such as reducing urine production and increasing water absorption in the kidneys, to prevent dehydration. Dry fasting must be carried out over specific periods, which only the dry fasting coach will be able to advise for each person, based on the study of the person's markers during the long dry fast and the Metatron NLS pre-cure bioresonance check-up.

Although dry fasting implies an absence of fluid consumption, the body has mechanisms for producing internal water via the breakdown of fats, which makes it possible to maintain functional hydration. It is important to understand that people who do dry fasting for more than 24 hours without supervision, without proper preparation and without understanding the mechanisms of dry fasting, and who take food supplements or unsuitable chemicals, may develop certain complications as a result of their dry fasting.

CHAPTER 3

Autophagy is the key therapeutic principle of fasting

Autophagy is a natural cellular mechanism by which the cells of our body degrade unnecessary or damaged components within the cell. This process helps to maintain the normal functioning (homeostasis) of the cell. The term 'autophagy' literally means 'eating yourself'. Although autophagy may give the impression of cellular destruction, it actually helps to eliminate harmful materials inside cells and revitalise them. Autophagy can completely destroy damaged molecules or recycle them into new components that can be used for cell repair.

In times of stress, when cells are deprived of nutrients or oxygen, autophagy can provide an alternative source of energy from recycled cell material to help them survive. Autophagy can also strengthen the immune system by eliminating toxins and infectious agents. Under certain conditions, autophagy can also induce programmed cell death (apoptosis). In short, autophagy is part of a cellular process that maintains homeostasis by striking a balance between the creation and degradation of cellular components.

1. The autophagy process

Autophagy is part of the metabolic process that helps cells convert food into a form of energy that cells can use to grow and divide. Metabolism balances two opposing activities: anabolism and catabolism. Anabolism is a process that synthesises molecules and builds cellular structures, while catabolism breaks them down. Autophagy is a catabolic process.

A human cell consists of a nucleus, itself surrounded by a semi-fluid substance called cytoplasm, enclosed in a cell membrane. The cytoplasm is made up of a solution called cytosol, protein molecules and specific structures called organelles, which are essential to the survival and functioning of the cell.

During autophagy, a semi-circular membrane called a phagophore forms and closes around certain molecules and organelles in the cytoplasm, becoming what is known as an autophagosome. The autophagosome fuses with an organelle called the lysosome. The lysosome contains digestive enzymes that break down the contents of the autophagosome. The resulting molecules are released into the cytosol to be recycled and used in the metabolic process.

Autophagy is a natural process that occurs constantly in the cell, less so when the cell is well nourished and more so during periods of stress. Autophagy can engulf non-specific cellular components or selectively eliminate damaged components or invasive bacteria and other pathogens.

2. The four most effective methods

1. **Dry fasting**. Fasting is one of the most effective methods of triggering autophagy. Intermittent and prolonged fasting can increase autophagic activity. A recent study indicates that time-restricted fasting improves markers of longevity and increases autophagy genes.

2. **Continuous calorie restriction.** Reducing your calories by ten to 40% of your usual requirements can also induce autophagy. Research shows that long-term calorie restriction is associated with an increase in autophagy

genes and levels of molecules involved in the elimination of damaged cells.

3. **Physical exercise.** Physical activity also induces autophagy in muscle tissue, particularly with high-intensity exercise. Autophagy markers increase immediately after short sessions of intense exercise and after prolonged sessions of moderate exercise.

4. **Consumption of polyphenols**. Polyphenols are plant compounds with health benefits. They can be found in foods or supplements and have been observed to trigger autophagy.

These strategies are effective in inducing autophagy, but it's important to choose the ones that suit you best.

1. Fasting for at least 16 hours: It is not entirely clear when autophagy begins during fasting, but fasting for at least 16 hours is generally recommended.
2. Consider prolonged fasting: It is possible that greater benefits of autophagy are obtained by fasting for prolonged periods of more than 24 hours of dry fasting.

3. Autophagy during fasting

Intermittent fasting is one way of inducing autophagy. Under normal conditions, when the cell has sufficient nutrients, autophagy degrades damaged components in the cell. When fasting deprives cells of nutrients, autophagy helps to digest certain cellular components to provide the energy needed for survival.

The liver stores excess glucose in the form of glycogen. When glucose levels fall during fasting, the liver converts the glycogen into glucose and releases it. After the stored glucose is used up, the liver breaks down fat to produce a substance called ketone, providing energy. This process is known as ketosis.

Many people follow intermittent fasting and calorie restriction diets to lose weight. A currently popular diet, known as the ketogenic diet, in which 75% of daily calories come from fat, is thought to induce ketosis and autophagy. However, there are few studies on the long-term effects of the ketogenic diet. Research indicates that intermittent fasting, calorie restriction and ketosis can trigger autophagy. However, most studies to date have only been carried out on animals. It is also unclear what type of cells trigger autophagy in response to fasting. For example, fasting can induce autophagy in different cells and not necessarily in fat cells.

4. How long do you have to fast to induce autophagy?

Depending on individual metabolism, significant autophagy may require two to four days of water fasting in humans and around 24 hours of dry fasting. Autophagy is thought to begin when glucose and insulin levels fall significantly. Animal studies have shown evidence of autophagy after 24 hours of fasting, peaking at around 48 hours of fasting. Some studies have detected autophagy in cultured human neutrophils (the most abundant type of immune cell in the blood) after 24 hours.

5. Benefits of autophagy

Autophagy has many benefits, not least anti-ageing. It can extend lifespan and maintain youthfulness by helping the body to function efficiently. That's why it's important to do dry fasting once or twice a year, which is the ideal frequency for maintaining health well into old age.

The benefits of autophagy, inside and outside cells:

- **Inside the cell:**

1. Reduces the oxidative stress that accelerates ageing.
2. Improves the conversion of nutrients into energy.
3. Helps eliminate waste and flush out toxins.
4. Breaks down damaged cells and proteins that can cause disease.
5. Recycles proteins into healthier versions.

- **Outside the cell:**

6. Reduces inflammation, a risk factor for many diseases.
7. Promotes skin cell renewal and the production of collagen and stem cells.
8. Improves hormonal balance.
9. Supports communication and nervous function.
10. Facilitates the elimination of ageing cells.

To reap these benefits, maintain optimal skin and age gracefully, there are ways of stimulating autophagy, notably through changes in diet and exercise.

6. Destruction of cysts, fibroids, mastoses, growths and diseased tissue

Dry fasting is the champion of abnormal cell destruction, as the body has the ability to self-heal and eliminate diseased tissues such as cysts, fibroids, tumours and other pathological growths. We will explore the biological mechanisms and effects of this unique fasting practice, while stressing the importance of approaching this method with caution and under competent supervision.

Autophagy is a natural cellular mechanism by which cells break down and recycle their own defective or useless components. During periods of fasting, especially in the total absence of food and water, autophagy activity intensifies, potentially allowing the elimination of damaged cells or accumulated pathological tissue, in response to poor lifestyle habits or somatisation processes.

The transition to ketosis metabolism triggered by fasting, where the body burns fat to produce energy in the absence of glucose, is suggested to have anti-inflammatory and cellular health-supporting effects. Theoretically, this metabolic transition during dry fasting could 'dry out' and help dissolve diseased tissue.

Before starting a fast, it is crucial to prepare the body, in particular by minimising toxaemia through a balanced diet and adequate hydration. The recommended duration for a dry fast to be effective in terms of autolysis of pathological tissues varies. However, periods of at least seven days are often recommended, with suggestions for repeating the cure after three to six months for optimum results.

Unlike surgical methods, which physically remove diseased tissue but may not eliminate the underlying causes of the disease and leave the body with a certain amount of toxaemia, autophagy-based dry fasting is envisaged as a non-invasive method of internal revitalisation. This prospect has given rise to debate within the medical community, which does not really want to investigate this therapeutic approach, as it is not profitable for Big Pharma. What's more, most doctors know nothing about it, apart from a few rare scholars. Dry fasting is more effective and safer than conventional treatments. Although dry fasting may offer an effective way of promoting health and treating certain pathologies, it is crucial to approach this practice with a full understanding of its implications.

7. The 2016 Nobel Prize in Medicine and autophagy

Deciphering the links between Yoshinori Ohsumi's discoveries and therapeutic prospects

In 2016, Yoshinori Ohsumi was awarded the Nobel Prize in Physiology or Medicine for his pioneering work on autophagy, a cellular process essential for the degradation and recycling of cellular components. This major advance not only broadened our fundamental understanding of cell biology, but also opened up new perspectives on how autophagy can be involved in therapeutic applications, particularly in the context of fasting.

- **Understanding Autophagy**

Autophagy is an evolutionarily inherited process that enables a cell to digest its own components. Prior to Ohsumi's work, the molecular mechanisms underlying autophagy were largely unknown. His research has made it possible to define the genes involved in this process and to understand how cells regulate autophagy to maintain their health and equilibrium.

- **Yoshinori Ohsumi's discoveries**

Ohsumi identified key proteins that orchestrate autophagy, demonstrating how cells form specialised structures called autophagosomes to engulf and degrade cellular components such as damaged proteins or unnecessary organelles. These discoveries have laid the foundations for research into autophagy, providing a framework for exploring its role in various pathological and physiological conditions.

- **Links with therapeutic fasting**

Although Ohsumi's findings are not directly related to fasting, links have been established between autophagy and metabolic conditions influenced by therapeutic fasting. For example, fasting can lower insulin levels and activate proteins such as AMP-activated protein kinase (AMPK), which are involved in regulating autophagy. These connections have led to growing interest in how fasting could be used to modulate autophagy for therapeutic purposes.

- **Therapeutic Perspectives**

The therapeutic implications of autophagy are vast. Research is underway to explore how modulation of this process could be exploited in the treatment of neurodegenerative diseases, metabolic diseases, cancers and other conditions. Therapeutic fasting is also emerging as a potential strategy for influencing autophagy in a clinical context.

Yoshinori Ohsumi's work has shed a brilliant light on autophagy, opening up new avenues in the understanding of fundamental cellular mechanisms. As therapeutic fasting and other metabolic approaches gain interest, the connection between Ohsumi's discoveries and clinical applications continues to evolve, promising an exciting future in medicine and biomedical research.

8. Autophagy specific to dry fasting

It is a fundamental survival mechanism that maintains cellular homeostasis by eliminating damaged or unnecessary components. The autophagy process begins with the formation of a membrane called the autophagosome, which encloses the cellular components to be degraded. The autophagosome then fuses with a lysosome, forming an autolysosome. Inside the autolysosome, enzymes break down the captured components into amino acids, lipids and other reusable molecules. Autophagy plays a crucial role in the regulation of metabolism, cell renewal, defence against infection and the prevention of neurodegenerative diseases.

1. **Activation of fasting signals**: When an individual goes into dry fasting, the body reacts by increasing the production of certain hormones, in particular adrenaline and glucagon, interferon and NK. These signals tell the cells that glucose reserves are exhausted and that it's time to switch to other sources of energy.
2. **Formation of autophagosomes**: Cells react by forming autophagosomes, membranes that encapsulate the cellular

components to be broken down. These autophagosomes act as cellular recycling bags.

3. **Fusion with lysosomes**: Autophagosomes then fuse with lysosomes, organelles containing enzymes capable of breaking down proteins, lipids and other cellular components into amino acids and other reusable elements.
4. **Recycling and regeneration:** Within the formed autolysosomes, broken down cellular components are transformed into usable materials, providing an alternative source of energy for the cells. This process contributes to cell regeneration and detoxification.

9. Potential benefits of autophagy during dry fasting

1. **Deep detoxification**: Dry fasting, by activating autophagy, can lead to deeper cellular detoxification than other forms of fasting. The cells break down toxins and damaged elements, helping to purify the body as a whole. Dry fasting is the royal fast.
2. **Cell renewal:** By eliminating defective cellular components, autophagy promotes cell renewal, offering even greater anti-ageing potential and increased regeneration than wet fasting.
3. **Stimulation of the immune system: By** activating autophagy, dry fasting strengthens the immune system by eliminating infected or damaged cells, thereby improving resistance to infection.

During dry fasting, the body undergoes significant metabolic changes which influence autophagy in several ways:

1. **Depletion of glycogen reserves:** When the body is deprived of food, it rapidly depletes its reserves of glycogen, the stored form of glucose. Once these reserves are depleted,

the body begins to use stored fat as a source of energy. This metabolic change can stimulate autophagy, as the breakdown of fat generates compounds that activate this process.

2. **Reduced insulin:** Fasting, particularly dry fasting, reduces insulin levels in the blood. A drop in insulin is associated with an increase in autophagy, as insulin normally inhibits this process.
3. **Activation of protein kinases**: During fasting, protein kinases such as AMP-activated protein kinase (AMPK) are activated. These proteins play a key role in regulating autophagy in response to variations in cellular energy levels.
4. **Increased levels of cAMP:** Fasting can also increase levels of cyclic adenosine monophosphate (cAMP), a cellular messenger. This increase can stimulate autophagy by modulating the activity of various proteins.
5. **Reduction in growth factors:** During fasting, levels of certain growth factors fall. This is the case for insulin-like growth factor 1 (IGF-1). These growth factors normally inhibit autophagy and their reduction during fasting may encourage this process.

Autophagy can play a beneficial role in cellular health by eliminating damaged components, promoting regeneration and protecting against certain diseases, including neurodegenerative diseases, cardiovascular disease and cancer. Autophagy, the cellular process of degrading and recycling damaged or superfluous cellular components, plays a crucial role in maintaining cellular health. Its involvement in the healing of human pathologies is complex and multifactorial. Here are some of the mechanisms by which autophagy can contribute to the therapeutic response to certain diseases:

1. **Elimination of protein aggregates:** Autophagy helps to eliminate abnormal protein aggregates, a common feature of many neurodegenerative diseases such as Alzheimer's

disease, Parkinson's disease and Huntington's disease. By eliminating these aggregates, autophagy can potentially slow the progression of these diseases.

2. **Degradation of damaged organelles:** Damaged cell organelles, such as defective mitochondria, can be degraded by autophagy. This process, known as mitophagy, helps to maintain the quality of cellular organelles and prevent the release of toxic molecules into the cell.
3. **Reduced inflammation**: Autophagy can reduce inflammation by eliminating elements that activate inflammatory pathways. Excessive inflammation is implicated in many diseases, including autoimmune diseases, cardiovascular disease and certain cancers.
4. **Suppression of uncontrolled cell proliferation:** In the case of cancer, autophagy can play a paradoxical role. On the one hand, it can promote the survival of cancer cells by supplying nutrients under conditions of stress. On the other hand, in certain circumstances, autophagy can help to inhibit uncontrolled cell proliferation by eliminating damaged cells.
5. **Metabolic regulation**: Autophagy can influence cellular metabolism, particularly in stressful situations such as dry fasting. It allows more efficient use of energy resources, which can be beneficial in the context of metabolic diseases such as diabetes.
6. **Improved response to infections**: Autophagy can help defend against infection by eliminating intracellular pathogens. It is an essential component of the intracellular immune response.

It is important to note that the involvement of autophagy in the healing of pathologies is a constantly evolving area of research. Although studies show promising links between autophagy and therapeutic response, further research is needed to fully understand how modulating this process could be used as a therapeutic approach in different pathological conditions.

CHAPTER 4

The mental aspect of dry fasting

Dry fasting is much more than a physical practice; it is a veritable mental and emotional expedition. More than simply abstaining from food and water, this process invites deep introspection and communion with the body, and requires mental preparation that is just as rigorous as the physical preparation. The mental state in which you undertake a dry fast is crucial: it can greatly influence the experience and the results obtained.

A positive approach, imbued with calm and serenity, makes fasting easier, allowing the body to concentrate on detoxification and regeneration. A tranquil mind allows you to listen more closely to your body, enabling you to fully experience each moment of fasting as a step towards profound transformation. It is therefore crucial to cultivate a state of inner well-being, acceptance and letting go.

On the other hand, a negative or stressful attitude can disrupt this delicate process. Negative emotions such as anxiety, anger or frustration consume precious energy, diverting internal resources that could be used for healing and revitalising the body. So it's essential not to allow yourself to be overwhelmed by disruptive thoughts and emotions, but rather to learn to observe them without judgement, to welcome them and let them pass.

To fully experience the transformative process of dry fasting, we recommend practising relaxation exercises such as meditation, yoga or conscious breathing. These practices help to refocus attention on the present moment, on bodily sensations, thereby encouraging a deep connection with oneself. They allow you to cultivate an attentive and caring presence towards your body, to identify and relieve physical or mental tensions, and to strengthen your ability to remain centred and serene in the face of the challenges of fasting.

It is also wise to avoid stressful or confrontational situations during the fast, whether professional or personal. Surrounding yourself with a calm and supportive environment, disconnecting from digital distractions and toxic social interactions, can go a long way towards maintaining positive energy and a focus on the healing process.

In short, dry fasting is an adventure that can be experienced both internally and externally. Preparing yourself mentally for this experience means giving yourself the means to get through this journey with grace and resilience, welcoming each stage as an opportunity for personal growth. By staying connected to your body, listening to your needs and cultivating a caring attitude towards yourself, fasting can become a source of transformation and renewal, paving the way to lasting well-being.

1. Get rid of your fears with dry fasting and rediscover your zest for life

Undertaking a dry fasting cure may initially arouse some doubts and apprehensions, which is perfectly natural. However, this approach offers a unique opportunity to face up to our fears, which are often unconscious, such as the fear of death, failure, pain, lack, or the fear of losing something or of things not being as they were before. To embark on dry fasting is to confront all these fears simultaneously. It is recognised that engaging in this process sooner or later leads to a form of liberation.

Beyond the immediate benefits of peace and relaxation experienced during fasting, there are also post-fasting benefits, when we reach a state of beneficial ketosis marked by abundant hormonal secretions. Dry fasting transports us into another dimension of time, where everything outside us seems to slow down. This state of consciousness, marked by deep introspection and pure awareness, is awakened from the start of the fast and lasts, enriched by numerous liberating benefits and sensations of release, for weeks or even months. It is also an intimate feeling of having achieved something positive for oneself, of having purified one's body and mind of many alienating influences.

Dry fasting encourages intimate communication with your inner self, opening the way to new perspectives, the exploration of new horizons and the exchange of ideas with other people seeking to evolve. After detoxifying and purifying your body, you'll be surprised by the flood of new ideas and energies that emerge, inspiring you to take action you might not have thought of before. This experience can lead to significant changes, breaking with elements of life that have become unsuitable, opening the door to a world of infinite possibilities.

Dry fasting invites you to reflect deeply on your existence, in a context of absolute deprivation, which can generate an interesting detachment from the superfluous and the material. Repeating the dry fasting cycles will take you through various emotional states: tears, crises, tension, pain, euphoria, pride, and finally a persistent joie de vivre despite the discomforts and challenges encountered. The benefits of hormesis, which are impressive and often unsuspected at first, can be seen at a profound level and are incomparable with juice diets or water fasts. Dry fasting is the therapy that will push you the furthest while giving you back the maximum benefits afterwards, provided it is well managed of course. In short, dry fasting is much more than a simple physical overhaul; it is a genuine inner therapy that encourages transcendence and the overall evolution of the human being.

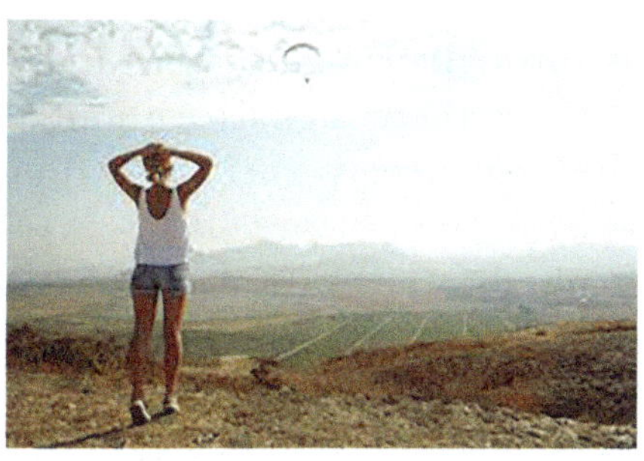

2. Dry fasting and pain management

Dry fasting, with its many virtues, can be a tricky road, especially when it comes to pain management. These pains, often perceived as elimination crises, are in reality signs of deep internal toxaemia.

During this period of dry fasting, every organ, tissue and muscle can undergo a profound renovation, where the old is eliminated to make way for the new. These transformations are not without consequences: the lack of water and sleep, coupled with an intensive cleansing of toxins, can cause significant discomfort. Toxins that have accumulated over time are expelled to the maximum, causing pain that can be intense. It is important to understand that although these pains can be severe, they are generally short-lived.

An elimination crisis does not last indefinitely. With dry fasting, these moments of intense pain are often followed by a marked improvement in symptoms, sometimes dramatic. This method is particularly effective in treating acute and inflammatory pain, thanks to the body's innate ability to initiate healing processes. It 's a life-saving mechanism, often unconscious, where the body's own vital force takes over to soothe and treat various ailments.

This healing process shows the extent to which the body possesses an intrinsic intelligence, capable of repairing itself. During a dry fast, the body mobilises this vital force to concentrate on eliminating toxins and repairing damaged tissue. This can be seen as a moment when the body speaks, indicating to us through pain the areas that need attention and care. Welcoming these signals without panic, but with understanding and patience, is crucial to getting through these elimination crises.

To accompany this process, it is advisable to practise relaxation and pain management techniques, such as meditation, deep breathing and everything else we offer during cures. These practices can help to reduce the intensity of pain and reinforce the feeling of well-being, despite temporary discomfort.

It is also essential to remember that each individual is unique and that reactions to dry fasting can vary greatly. Listening carefully to your body and, if possible, being accompanied by a healthcare professional experienced in conducting dry fasts, can greatly contribute to a safe and rewarding experience.

In short, the pain experienced during a dry fast, although sometimes intense, is evidence of a profound healing process. They indicate that the body is actively working to rid itself of harmful elements and regenerate itself. Embracing this experience with patience and confidence in your own body's ability to heal can transform dry fasting into a profoundly transformative and beneficial experience.

3. Sweet cravings before or after dry fasting

Sugar is one of the greatest health hazards, acting like a poison or an anaesthetic drug that is hard to get rid of completely. Nevertheless, it is possible to try to reduce your intake or to ingest it in a less harmful way, for example after a hearty meal of vegetables.

Sugar, which is omnipresent in our modern diet, is at the root of many health problems. Excessive consumption is associated with a variety of pathologies, including obesity, type 2 diabetes, cardiovascular disease, certain cancers, deteriorating dental health and it can even influence mental health by promoting anxiety and depression. It creates an addiction similar to that of drugs, leading to increased consumption. What's more, it causes repeated insulin spikes which, over the long term, can lead to insulin resistance, the prelude to diabetes. From a metabolic point of view, over-consumption leads to an accumulation of fat, increasing the risk of chronic diseases.

Dry fasting is an effective strategy for countering the harmful effects of sugar on health. By temporarily eliminating food intake, fasting allows the body to draw on its glucose and fat reserves, encouraging a metabolic reset. This helps to regulate insulin levels and reduce resistance to this hormone, offering protection against type 2 diabetes. Dry fasting also helps to detoxify the body, eliminating accumulated toxins, including those resulting from the breakdown of sugars.

Intermittent fasting, alternating periods of fasting and restricted food windows, is particularly well suited to changing eating habits and reducing sugar dependency. This practice teaches the body to manage its energy reserves and optimise the use of glucose, having a positive influence on weight and body composition, promoting fat loss while preserving muscle mass.

To reap the full benefits of dry fasting in the fight against the damaging effects of sugar, it is advisable to combine it with a balanced diet, rich in essential nutrients, favouring whole foods while limiting added sugars and ultra-processed foods as much as possible. Adopting an active lifestyle and managing stress are also crucial to reinforcing the positive effects of fasting on metabolic health.

However, it is important to note that when resuming eating after a dry fast, it is advisable to maintain ketosis for at least a week and to avoid sugars or processed products for two months. This period constitutes a significant test to evaluate the management of this restriction. When the diet is resumed, it is important to avoid pitfalls such as sugary drinks, cakes, chocolate with less than 70% cocoa, and excess carbohydrates (pasta, bread, rice and other starchy foods), which can have a negative impact on blood sugar levels. The real indicator is the glycated haemoglobin level (HbA1c), which reflects the average blood sugar level over three months. A level above 5.5 indicates pre-diabetes, requiring an urgent dietary change.

When I discovered the protocol for exiting dry fasting in Russia, I realised that it contained a number of errors. First and foremost, it is important to continue in ketosis with food recovery and not to bring in any sugar. Liquid Russian compote is a major mistake, as is the fruit given from day two, whether watermelon or apples. The same goes for kefir, honey and buckwheat. Personally, I've seen bouts of gluttony in people who very quickly resume their sweet cravings from the second day onwards, as if to compensate for all the sugar they hadn't eaten during the week. What's more, I don't agree with the three meals a day proposed by the Russian school. The fodmap diet and the absence of carbohydrates should really be applied for at least one week after recovery, or even longer for those who want to get the maximum benefit from their therapeutic dry fasting.

4. What to say to those around you who are dry fasting and with whom?

When you're considering dry fasting, communicating with those around you about it requires thought and tact. If you choose to fast alone, you have a certain amount of freedom in that you don't have to answer to anyone. However, if you decide to talk to others about it, be prepared for a variety of reactions. Some people may judge you negatively or question your approach, while others may offer you support and encouragement.

Undertaking dry fasting with your family presents particular challenges. The difficulty lies in the fact that it is less easy to detach yourself completely, as you will constantly have to interact with your loved ones who may worry when they see you tired. This situation can prevent you from achieving the depth of fasting you need for optimal regeneration. The pressure of having to look strong in front of your family can also push you into overdrive. What's more, managing the return to food in this environment can be energy-consuming, diverting precious resources that would otherwise be used for post-fasting regeneration.

I strongly recommend getting out of your daily routine and considering fasting in a new environment. This approach encourages change and supports your inner transformation, while facilitating the adoption of new healthy lifestyle habits.

Fasting in an urban environment can be counter-productive. In a context of dry fasting, the absence of water intake makes the body more receptive to its environment, including oxygen, humidity and pollution. As a result, you run the risk of assimilating harmful elements present in urban air.

Taking part in a professionally supervised dry fasting group can be a liberating experience. Such a setting eliminates daily constraints and encourages total letting go. It provides a safe space to express and share tensions, pain, tears and emotions, without fear of judgement. Sharing experiences within the group can greatly contribute to your inner healing process. What's more, the motivation and mutual support within the group make the dry fasting journey much easier. The treatments and biotherapies available on site can increase the effectiveness of fasting, while the conviviality of the group brings a dimension of joy and enriching sharing.

In my personal experience, dry fasts carried out in a group have always been more impactful and beneficial than those carried out in solitude. The group dynamic and professional supervision create an environment conducive to a profound and transformative fasting experience. In my experience, I also advise against fasting in groups of people doing water fasts or juice and broth-based diets. You'll be completely out of step with them, and they really won't understand what you're doing and why you're doing it. What's more, you'll see people who don't have the same approach or the same energy as those who practise dry fasting. You'll hear them talking about everything and nothing, while you yourself will be going through a rich and intense inner experience. I explain all this because I've been through it myself and it confirmed to me that it was preferable not to try this experience again, that it was better to be alone or to be with dry fasters.

CHAPTER 5

Emergencies and acute crises in dry fasting

In the field of medicine and health, there is a constant search for effective solutions for treating emergencies and acute crises. Among the approaches revisited in the light of ancestral practices and alternative medicine, dry fasting is emerging as a promising method, offering a natural and powerful response to these critical situations.

1. The basics of dry fasting in emergency situations

Acute attacks, whether caused by illness, infection or pain, are often the result of an accumulation of toxins, stress and a harmful diet. These often multifactorial factors generate an exacerbated inflammatory reaction within the body. Dry fasting, with its radical approach, is a first response to these emergencies.

By imitating the instinctive behaviour of animals who rest and fast to overcome illness or injury, dry fasting induces a state in which the body can concentrate fully on healing itself. This ancient practice is based on the principle that in the absence of food and fluids, the body draws on its reserves and intrinsic capacities to regenerate itself.

2. The benefits of dry fasting in an emergency

- **Inflammation reduction**: Dry fasting helps to reduce inflammation levels in the body, offering relief in emergency situations where inflammation is an aggravating factor.

- **Reduced pain**: By modulating the inflammatory response, dry fasting can also reduce the sensation of pain, making emergency management more comfortable.
- **Conservation of vital energy**: By avoiding digestion, which is often energy-consuming, dry fasting allows vital energy to be redirected towards the body's repair and healing processes.
- **Prevention of worsening**: By limiting the intake of substances that can add to the body's toxic burden, dry fasting helps to prevent any worsening of the state of health.
- **Facilitating post-operative recovery**: Used in preparation for surgery and during the convalescence period, dry fasting can speed up recovery and wound healing.

3. Why dry fasting in an emergency?

The key to recovery in the event of an emergency lies in the individual's vitality. Children, for example, recover quickly from crises because of their high vitality, capable of expelling waste and toxins at an accelerated rate. By preserving this vital energy, dry fasting facilitates the healing process.

Dry fasting is a revolutionary approach to the treatment of emergencies, offering a natural and effective alternative to conventional methods. By encouraging the body's self-regulation and intrinsic healing, this practice revives ancestral knowledge, while opening up new ways of understanding and managing acute crises in modern medicine.

CHAPTER 6

Dry fasting and rejuvenation

1. Mechanisms

Dry fasting increases metabolic processes such as autophagy, stem cell regeneration and human growth hormone, recycling old cells and creating new ones, a process that renews your whole body and slows down ageing.

This method of dry fasting, described as miraculous, has been recommended by many religions throughout history as a way of resetting our health. Calorie restriction has long been linked to longevity. It is only recently that the anti-ageing benefits of fasting have become widely recognised, mainly thanks to the growing popularity of intermittent water fasting but also to practitioners of dry fasting.

However, dry fasting is the undisputed champion of all self-induced anti-ageing efforts. Dry fasting offers all the benefits of water fasting in just a third of the time required for water fasting. The metabolic processes that generally begin after three days (72 hours) of prolonged water fasting begin in just one day (24 hours) of dry fasting.

Between 12 and 24 hours of dry fasting, the reduction in sugar and water consumption triggers a massive change in your body's main source of fuel. It's as if your car has just switched from diesel to electric.

Your body now runs on a clean, superior energy called ketones: a chemical substance that replaces glucose or sugar as the fuel source for your cells. Ketones, or the state of ketosis, and other factors of dry fasting, trigger metabolic changes resulting from an internal recycling process, mainly induced by processes such as autophagy, stem cell regeneration and the secretion of human growth hormone.

Firstly, autophagy allows the consumption of unhealthy, useless, old, diseased and damaged cells, leaving only the healthiest to survive. Stem cell regeneration and proliferation increase during dry fasting, dividing and creating new cells to fill the void left by diseased cells degraded by autophagy.

Human growth hormone (HGH) increases, stimulating blood circulation, improving sleep and brain function, reducing body fat and increasing the growth of collagen and lean muscle mass.

This metabolic renewal rejuvenates all the vital cells, tissues and systems in your body, including your vascular system. Your vascular age is the age of your heart, arteries and blood vessels. Vascular age can be influenced by many factors and is higher if you are a smoker, drinker with a poor lifestyle, have high cholesterol or if there is a history of heart problems in the family. This is why some people appear much older than their biological age, and why heart attacks can occur suddenly in someone in their thirties.

The body is an intelligent organism and knows what it needs most for its well-being. Your vascular system is vital to your overall health, which means it gets a golden treatment. A cleaning service during dry fasting removes all the old, damaged cells and improves blood vessels, arteries and heart tissue, giving you new walls and a fresh coat of paint to be stronger, healthier and younger.

2. Dry fasting and apoptosis

Another important source of rejuvenation is apoptosis, a programmed cell death mechanism. Most cells in the human body live actively for a few years, then age and become functionally passive, as is the case with fat cells. Even colonies of micro-organisms have a mechanism for 'food recycling' of ageing cells. All multicellular organisms use their old cells as a source of raw materials and energy, as a reserve in case of emergency.

When the 'dietary recycling' mechanism remains inactive for a prolonged period, these old cells can become a factory of pathological proteins attacking their own immune system. These factors disrupt central and tissue regulation, meaning they become progenitor cells for malignant tumours. They must therefore be eliminated from the body. For millions of years, periods of forced fasting have been the norm in animal life. For multicellular organisms, the process of eliminating useless, structurally or functionally atypical cells has never been a problem.

Apoptosis, or programmed cell death, is incorporated into the genetic apparatus of all multicellular organisms – animals, plants and fungi – and is an energy-dependent and genetically controlled process. It is activated by specific signals and aims to free the body of weak, useless or altered cells. Around 5% of the body's cells undergo apoptosis every day, with new cells taking their place during the process. The cell disappears without a trace in 15 to 120 minutes.

Apoptosis is one of the basic mechanisms of oncological self-prevention. Excessive apoptotic activity can lead to cell loss disorders, aplasia, degenerative processes and tissue defects and malformations. Conversely, deficient apoptosis can lead to uncontrolled cell growth, a mechanism underlying cancer, autoimmune processes and premature ageing. For example, there is good reason to believe that excessive apoptosis is associated with serious diseases such as aplastic anaemia, amyotrophic lateral sclerosis, Alzheimer's disease, AIDS, etc.

Global changes occur during dry fasting. On the one hand, the physiological process of apoptosis is invigorated and improved: the body renews and rejuvenates itself at the expense of the death of old, diseased or altered cells. Secondly, the pathological mechanisms of apoptosis are eliminated: premature ageing, neoplasms, etc.

Let's analyse these mechanisms in detail. Understood as a community of cells, the organism during dry fasting 'eats' not only fat cells, but also all superfluous, morbid or defective elements. The organism's continued existence is impossible without the self-cleansing function of its cell populations. Cells infected by viruses, toxins or damaged by radiation, as well as those that have reached their biological limit, have one thing in common: they must leave the organism or be eaten. This happens in nature.

In the absence of external nutrition, a particular type of signalling molecule appears within a multicellular organism. These molecules activate intracellular proteins in the cytoplasm of atypical cells. Cells that do not participate in the collective activity of the organism are sensitive and respond to these molecules by triggering a self-destruction mechanism: the cell "shuts down" all its programmes, its nucleus "contracts" and begins to subdivide. Without destroying its outer envelope, the cell subdivides into five to ten "apoptotic bodies" and is absorbed by other cells. This is what happens in a colony of micro-organisms. Otherwise, it is digested in the intestine, sharing the fate of fat cells.

3. Can dry fasting make you look younger?

Your skin represents between 10 and 20% of your total body weight, making it the largest organ in the body. Dry fasting triggers metabolic processes that eliminate old cells and replace them with healthier, younger ones. Since the skin is an external indicator of internal well-being, it also looks younger.

The reduction in skin elasticity and plumpness results from the loss of two major proteins: collagen and elastin. During a dry fast, the cellular recycling mechanism of autophagy eliminates all unhealthy proteins and cells, leaving only the healthiest and most vital cells.

As a result of the proliferation of stem cells, more fibroblasts are generated to further increase collagen production in the skin, eliminating fine lines and wrinkles.

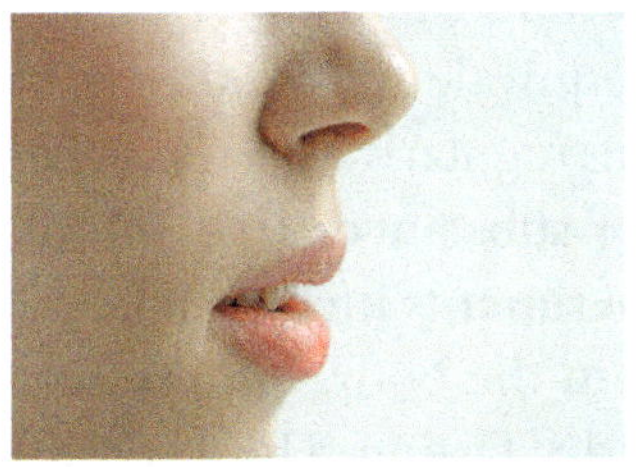

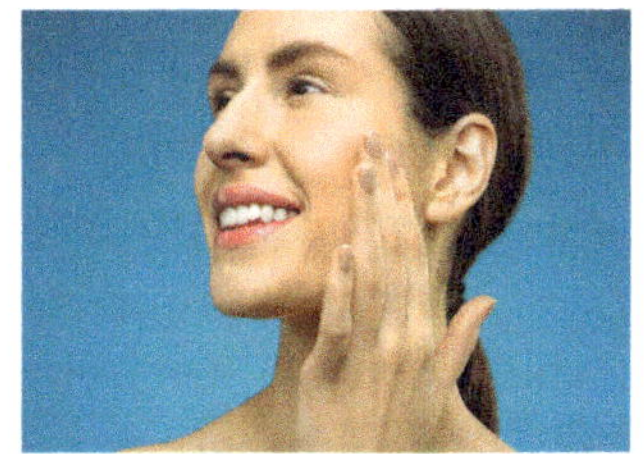

Human growth hormone (HGH) is also secreted into the system. HGH increases collagen production, tightening the skin while reducing fat and increasing muscle mass, which can help tone sagging skin, making it look younger. Research has shown that HGH also makes skin thicker. HGH also improves sleep, combating a significant reason for poor skin health.

4. Can dry fasting reverse ageing?

Theoretically, by fasting regularly, eliminating unwanted cells and creating new immortal stem cells capable of regenerating into any cell in the body, it would be possible to reverse ageing. By making frequent use of the mechanisms of dry fasting and a healthy lifestyle, there is even the possibility of living forever. Scientific experiments have been conducted to prove this theory, such as a study on mice that reversed wrinkles and hair loss, and a study on worms that lived up to six times longer after fasting.

Numerous experiments on lower life forms strongly indicate that fasting prolongs life and improves quality of life. Professor M. Child of the University of Chicago has studied insects which normally live for three to four weeks, but which, when subjected to a reduction in their diet and fasting, remained active and young for three to four years.

Suren Arakeylan (1928-2002) conducted an experiment on caged hens that had stopped laying eggs but resumed laying after fasting. Another experiment tested hens that had fasted. While the average hen lives for six years, those that fasted lived to

18 years, with one in particular reaching 21 years. For a human being, this life extension would be equivalent to 250 years!

Given that not eating or drinking regularly may not be viable, science is exploring the creation of substances that mimic the effects of extreme fasting. Some experiments include a ketogenic diet, where ketones are used as fuel in the body, but this method will never have the effectiveness of dry fasting. However, it does allow you to do something worthwhile for your health.

5. Can dry fasting improve skin quality?

Loose or sagging skin is the result of a variety of factors, from ageing to lifestyle to extreme weight loss. However, the loss of skin tone and bounce is mainly down to a reduction in collagen, elastin and, overall, unhealthy skin cells, reflecting the overall health of the body. As dry fasting stimulates autophagy, the body breaks down and 'consumes' superfluous proteins, organelles and cellular structures. This process also targets unhealthy skin cells, as the skin is a significant organ.

Distinctions are observed between previously obese individuals who have lost weight through fasting and those who have lost weight through calorie restriction or dieting. In most cases, prolonged water fasting or dry fasting allows the body to eliminate excess skin. The increase in stem cells induced by dry fasting also generates new proteins, such as elastin and collagen, to improve skin health. This proliferation of new healthy cells stimulates the production of fibroblasts, supporting the growth of collagen. At the same time, elastin, a connective tissue, is actively produced, giving our skin that delicious elasticity, promoting resilience and a rapid return to its original shape. Human growth hormone will also help to firm the skin, strengthening it and encouraging increased production of collagen, for firmer skin.

By promoting autophagy, dry fasting induces the consumption of excess proteins, organelles and cellular structures. This process also extends to the elimination of unhealthy skin cells, recognising the skin's crucial role as a major organ. This increase in the proliferation of healthy cells also stimulates the production of fibroblasts, supporting the growth of collagen. Human growth hormone also helps to firm the skin, reinforcing its structure and boosting collagen production, ultimately giving your skin a firmer appearance.

6. Increased rejuvenation power of dry fasting compared to wet fasting

This is because diseased, degenerated and weakened cells cannot cope with the extreme conditions imposed by dry fasting. When cells evolve in a comfortable environment, they become accustomed to a constant level of nutrients and water, losing the ability to renew and reinvigorate themselves effectively. It's as if they become lazy in triggering tissue self-renewal mechanisms.

However, as soon as food and water stop entering the gastrointestinal tract, new conditions of existence are established in the body. Under these conditions, the old biomolecules are "dismantled", unstable cells die and decompose, and the deficit in energetic and plastic substances is compensated for at their expense. But at the same time, new cells are synthesised that are more resistant and capable of surviving the new circumstances.

7. Dry fasting and the anti-ageing effect

Why is the rejuvenating effect on the body greater during dry fasting than with water fasting? Sick, degenerated and weak cells cannot withstand extreme conditions; they die and decompose. Which remain? Cells with good organisation and extensive, efficient genetic engineering, because those that are not affected survive and maintain their functions.

Fasting helps to get rid of useless, weak, sick and harmful parasitic cells. They do not perform their functions and it is preferable to eliminate them in time, without allowing them to die a natural death, otherwise they could generate a progeny of weaker, inoperative cells. After dry fasting, the strong cells remain, which divide to produce high-quality daughter cells with the same properties as the mother cells.

Dry fasting can stimulate autophagy to a higher level than water fasting. In the total absence of food and fluids, the body can intensify its cellular cleansing mechanisms to eliminate damaged or unnecessary cellular components.

- Some people report that dry fasting can help to control appetite better than water fasting. The total absence of food and fluids can create a feeling of satiety that lasts longer, which helps those seeking to regulate their calorie intake.
- Dry fasting can stimulate the metabolism in a unique way. The absence of fluids can induce a more intense metabolic response, encouraging more efficient use of energy reserves.
- During dry fasting, there is a concentration of electrolytes, as no water is consumed. Some claim that this concentration can have beneficial effects on electrolyte balance and cellular function, although this requires careful monitoring to avoid any imbalance.
- The absence of liquids during dry fasting can potentially reduce water retention and bloating, making some people feel lighter.

8. Growth hormone system: interactions with the skin

Guilherme Póvoa 1, Lucia Martins Diniz Affiliations
https://www.scielo.br/j/abd/a/Jx65WTSSM4rdG6yxwDL4zgR/?lang=pt

Summary

This article describes the growth hormone system, focusing on its possible effects on epidermal cells, dermal structures and wound healing. A literature review was carried out on studies concerning the growth hormone molecule, its receptor and carrier proteins, as well as other proteins involved in the mechanisms of its manifestation in dermal tissues.

Dry fasting and body energy.

Water stands out as an exceptional carrier of energetic information. This astonishing property stems from water's distinctive molecular composition and the variability of its cluster structure. Scientific evidence supports the idea that long before symptoms of illness appear, local zones of 'heavy' water or water with an irregular structure, which can be described as pathological zones, form in the human body. These zones, which incubate negative energies such as curses, harbour harmful forces. During a dry fast, the body orchestrates the replacement of the old 'dead' water with high quality, energetically renewed and 'living' water, synthesised internally. Dry fasting, often perceived as a deprivation of organic food, does not deplete energy. On the contrary, it draws on the subtle energy of the surrounding environment. This subtle energy is used more intensely after dry fasting, creating a hyperactive restorative effect. Even more surprisingly, dry fasting emerges as a very intense spiritual undertaking, purifying the soul and body, strengthening the will and nurturing a positive state of mind in the early stages of personal evolution.

The benefits of dry fasting extend beyond purely physiological improvements. Perceptive abilities undergo a significant increase, with tactile senses, skin sensitivity and sense of smell reaching heightened levels, revealing interesting effects. This heightened awareness makes it possible to discern the freshness of an egg or detect the presence of preservatives in food without direct contact.

During dry fasting, sweat secretion decreases and the skin changes from a secreter to an absorber. This change means that substances can be absorbed by touch, or even tasted in the mouth. Intuition intensifies, similar to an increased perception of energy zones, sometimes manifesting itself in the form of telepathic abilities specific to each individual.

Those who practise dry fasting on a regular basis demonstrate a strengthened willpower. Abstinence from food for 24 hours a week cultivates mental strength, paving the way for sound decision-making and firm determination in the face of life's challenges. During my practice, I have seen profound transformations in people who have become the best versions of themselves.

The positive transformations after dry fasting are not limited to perception and mental resilience. Physical changes include improved resistance to cold, reversal of grey hair, a slimming effect, improved vision, clearer eyes, cessation of snoring and improved breathing quality. Dental improvements abound, from the disappearance of yellow tartar to firmer gums.

In addition, dry fasting is associated with the resolution of persistent health problems such as hypertension, insomnia and chronic runny nose. In summary, while many health benefits can be achieved through various fasting methods, dry fasting stands out for its effectiveness and faster results. It is becoming a holistic approach, not only for physical regeneration, but also for spiritual, physical and mental renewal, making it a first-level therapy.

CHAPTER 7

Is dry fasting effective for weight loss?

1. The little-known dangers of sugar and fructose for the liver

Sugar, present in many of the foods and drinks we consume every day, is often underestimated in terms of its health risks. Among the different types of sugar, fructose, which is found in large quantities in high-fructose corn syrups and fruit, presents particular challenges for our bodies.

Unlike glucose, another type of sugar, fructose is mainly metabolised by the liver. When we consume fructose in excess, the liver becomes overloaded and converts a large proportion of the fructose into fat. This excessive conversion can lead to an accumulation of fat in the liver, known as non-alcoholic fatty liver disease. This disorder can progress to more serious complications such as cirrhosis and liver failure.

2. Dirtying the body and weight gain

Excess sugar in the diet is not just a liver problem. It affects the whole body. Excess fructose transformed into fat by the liver is released into the bloodstream, contributing to an increase in triglycerides, a type of blood fat. This in turn can lead to an increased risk of cardiovascular disease.

What's more, sugar, particularly fructose, can disrupt the body's satiety signals, leading to overeating. Foods rich in sugar tend to be less satiating, leading to higher calorie consumption. This over-consumption contributes significantly to weight gain and obesity, a major health problem in many societies.

To minimise the health risks associated with excessive sugar consumption, a number of strategies can be adopted:

1. Reduce consumption of sugary drinks and processed foods, which are often major sources of added sugar, particularly fructose.
2. Increase your consumption of whole fruit rather than fruit juice, as the fibre present in whole fruit helps to moderate the absorption of fructose.
3. Keep an eye on nutrition labels to become more aware of the hidden sources of sugar in everyday foods.
4. Increase the ratio of fats and animal proteins, which will make you less tempted to eat other things.

In conclusion, although sugar can add a pleasant flavour to our food, it is crucial to be aware of its potentially harmful effects on our health, particularly with regard to the metabolism of fructose by the liver and the consequences of over-consumption of sugar on our weight and general well-being.

3. Weight loss through dry fasting: an effective, natural method

This approach, which relies on the use of body reserves for energy, has a number of advantages for those looking to lose weight in a healthy and sustainable way.

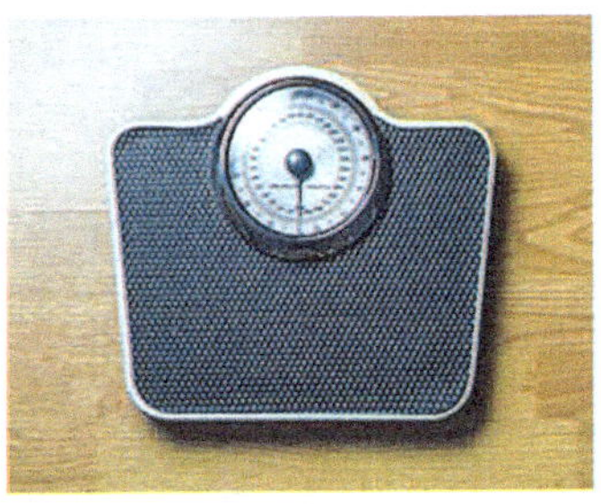

How does dry fasting work for weight loss?

1. **Stimulation of lipolysis.** Dry fasting accelerates lipolysis, the process by which the body breaks down stored fat to produce energy. In the absence of food and water, the body turns to its fat reserves, resulting in effective weight loss.
2. **Elimination of toxins.** This method also promotes detoxification. Toxins stored in fatty tissue are released and eliminated, contributing to better overall health.
3. **Reduced inflammation and oedema.** Dry fasting helps to relieve inflammation and oedema, often associated with obesity and weight-related health problems.

Benefits of dry fasting for weight loss

- **Fast, effective weight loss.** Many dry fasters report rapid and significant weight loss.
- **No constant feeling of hunger.** Unlike some diets, dry fasting reduces the sensation of hunger after the initial adaptation phases.
- **Improved skin condition.** Unlike other weight-loss methods, the skin does not generally become flabby or loose after weight loss by dry fasting.
- **Overall improvement in health.** Participants often observe an improvement in their general well-being, with benefits such as lower blood pressure, better digestion and less strain on the heart.

Precautions and recommendations

- **Therapeutic follow-up.** Before starting dry fasting, it is essential to consult a health professional, especially if you have any pre-existing medical problems.
- **Duration of fasting.** The duration of dry fasting should be adapted to the individual, starting with short periods and gradually increasing under supervision.
- **Eating again**. The period of resumption of eating after fasting is crucial. It is advisable to reintroduce food gradually, favouring a healthy, balanced diet to maintain the benefits of fasting.
- **Slimming effect:** during dry fasting, the body receives neither food nor water, so there is no external supply of energy. The body is forced to produce energy and water endogenously, i.e. internally. For this reason, unusual chemical reactions begin to occur in the body and metabolic processes are altered. For example, less muscle tissue is lost than fat tissue.

During water fasting, muscle and fat tissue are reduced in roughly proportion. However, during dry fasting, the patient acts as a water saver. This is because the body maintains its vital capacity at the expense of reserve fat. The adipose tissue is destroyed very effectively and does not regain its initial volume, and the adipocytes are attacked. In fact, it is destroyed three to four times faster than muscle tissue, because adipose tissue is more than 90% water, whereas muscle tissue remains relatively intact. The body does not suffer from a lack of water, as it obtains the water it needs from adipose tissue. During dry fasting, adipose tissue burns three times faster than during water fasting. Burnt fat reserves are not restored, unlike during water fasting. Fat deposits are digested earlier and better than during water fasting. After a water fast, adipose tissue is restored more quickly, especially when you resume the same diet as before the fast. With dry fasting, this happens to a lesser extent. Nutrition based on the body's own reserves is perfectly balanced. The body only takes what it needs from its reserves, rather than what is artificially imposed from outside.

To sum up, as well as a long dry fast, you need to include a dietary adjustment to reduce insulin secretion as much as possible. This means a drastic reduction in carbohydrates and fruit. Make sure you get enough sleep, reduce stress and take regular exercise, all key factors in maintaining a stable weight.

CHAPTER 8

The different types of dry fasting

1. Description of operation

Water fasting, with a normal intake of water, is the most commonly used form of fasting in clinical practice because it has been the most extensively studied. Dry fasting is relatively recent and little known at present, and therefore little studied.

From a physiological point of view, during dry fasting, the body does not suffer from a fluid deficit because each kilogram of lipid mass (glycogen) releases up to one litre of endogenous (metabolic) water. At normal room temperature, the body does not lose large quantities of fluids through perspiration from the lungs and skin: around 1.5 litres a day. So the water deficit never exceeds 0.5 litres per day, physiologically acceptable values in conditions of reduced basic metabolism.

The practice of dry fasting recommends short dry fasting exercises (one to three days), during which neither enemas nor laxatives are prescribed. During dry fasting, the typical fasting phases are reduced. The food excitement phase lasts only a few hours. The phase of increased ketosis lasts from one to three days. Observation shows that the division of fat deposits begins earlier and is more complete. In addition, a high concentration of biologically active substances such as hormones, immunocompetent cells and immunoglobulins is detected in the body fluids. Contrary to popular belief, 'dry' fasting is objectively better tolerated than 'wet' fasting. Moreover, in cases of illnesses such as bronchial asthma, hypertension or forms of allergy, a three-day dry fast has been shown to be much more effective than a three-day wet fast. Based on the studies and results obtained, we can say that three days of absolute or dry fasting correspond to seven to nine days of water fasting.

Combined fasting refers to absolute (dry) fasting and (water) fasting. This is a method of consecutive application of absolute (dry) fasting for two to three days, followed by wet fasting for ten to 14 days. Under this practice, we advise patients to abstain from food and water for one to three days (depending on individual tolerance) and no cleansing procedure (enemas) is prescribed. From the second to the fourth day, patients begin to take water at a dose of ten to 12 mg per kg of body weight per day, allowing the process to continue with wet fasting. Some researchers have observed that the use of combined fasting enables peak acidity to be reached more quickly and body fat to be reduced considerably. In the treatment of hypertensive patients, normalisation of blood pressure begins earlier, thereby reducing the time needed for fasting and, consequently, the length of time patients spend in hospital. This method is the preferred alternative in cases of obesity or oedema as a complication of the main disease.

In addition, the combination of dry and wet fasting is well tolerated by patients. It has a therapeutic effect even in cases where the overall duration is reduced, and optimises the course of therapy thanks to the early onset of the acidotic crisis.

- **Disadvantages**

During combined fasting, there is no elimination of "endogenous heavy dead water" from the body. The anti-inflammatory effect is less pronounced compared with the same effect during dry fasting, and the depurative effect is also weaker. To achieve a positive therapeutic effect, a long period of water fasting of at least 30 days is required. The problem is that it then takes months to recover and build up minerals again. This is not the case with dry fasting, where vitality returns fairly quickly. Diets based on juices and broths, such as Buchinger's, are not real fasts. The one-week cures on offer everywhere are mainly commercial and have no major therapeutic effect, apart from a bit of digestive rest and a slight detox. This type of business is very much in vogue, however, because the marketing is well developed. Participants take part in daily physical activity without any problems. But this greatly reduces autophagy, as all nervous energy is allocated to physical activity to the detriment of physiological renewal. What's more, this type of cure poses no specific difficulties for those accompanying the patient, as curative crises are virtually non-existent. There aren't too many symptoms for the cure leader to deal with.

With combined fasting, it is advisable to start strictly with dry fasting days and then continue with water fasting. It is dangerous to reverse the practice and do the opposite, because it is always absolutely necessary to start with the process that imposes a more extreme modality, and then move on to a modality which is more acceptable to the body.

There are two types of dry fasting. The first is gentle fasting with an affusion of ice-cold water at less than 11 degrees, i.e. a bucket of cold water on the head twice a day. The second is strict dry fasting, with no contact with water.

Fasting with rinsing the mouth, brushing the teeth, taking a hot shower or bath is not considered to be true dry fasting. However, as there is a reduction in water intake, some beneficial effects may nevertheless occur, but this type of fasting is less effective than strict fasting.

Dry fasting triggers a series of complex metabolic and physiological reactions in the body. During the first few hours, the body goes through several key stages to adapt to the absence of food and water intake. Here's an overview of what happens in the body during this time, focusing on the processes of glycolysis, gluconeogenesis and autophagy.

0-24 hours: Initial changes

- **Glycolysis and glycogen utilisation.** As mentioned above, the body depends on glycolysis and the breakdown of glycogen for energy.
- **Initial hormonal responses.** There is a slight increase in growth hormone (GH) to promote lipolysis and preserve muscle mass at the start of fasting.

24-48 hours: Activation of gluconeogenesis

- **Increased gluconeogenesis**. The body intensifies glucose production from non-carbohydrate sources.
- **Increase in GH, the growth hormone.** The production of GH or growth hormone continues to increase, facilitating lipolysis and helping to maintain muscle mass and metabolic function. GH also helps to stimulate cell repair and growth during dry fasting.

48-72 hours: Increase in ketogenesis and autophagy

- **Ketogenesis:** The body produces ketone bodies at an increased rate, providing an alternative energy source for the brain and other organs.
- **Autophagy and BDNF.** Activation of autophagy cleans cells of damaged components. During this phase, production of BDNF may also increase, promoting neuronal health, neurogenesis and brain plasticity. BDNF is essential for learning, memory and mood regulation.

After 72 hours: Profound metabolic and hormonal adaptations

- **Prolonged metabolic adaptations.** The body adapts to make efficient use of ketone bodies and glucose for energy, minimising muscle protein breakdown.

- **Sustained increase in GH or growth hormone and BDNF.** GH production remains high, supporting lipolysis, muscle protein preservation and cell regeneration. Increased levels of BDNF contribute to neuronal resilience and may improve cognitive function.
- **Other hormones.** Hormonal adaptations also include adjustments in insulin, cortisol and adrenaline levels, all of which play a role in energy management, stress response and metabolic regulation during fasting.

These hormonal and metabolic changes show how the body adapts to maintain homeostasis and promote survival in the absence of food and water intake. GH and BDNF play crucial roles in preserving muscle mass, promoting metabolic health and neuronal protection, highlighting the potential long-term health benefits of fasting. Nevertheless, it is essential to remember that dry fasting can involve risks, particularly when practised for prolonged periods without competent supervision.

After 72 hours of dry fasting, the body enters a more advanced phase of fasting where profound metabolic and physiological adaptations occur to maintain homeostasis in the absence of water and nutrient intake. At this stage, the body's survival mechanisms are fully engaged to optimise the use of energy reserves and preserve vital functions.

Metabolic adaptations

- **Increased ketogenesis.** The body increases the production of ketone bodies to provide an alternative energy source to glucose for the brain and other tissues. This marks a significant shift in energy metabolism, from dependence on glucose to increased use of ketone bodies.
- **Reduced gluconeogenesis.** Although gluconeogenesis continues to supply glucose from non-carbohydrate sources (such as amino acids and glycerol), the

efficiency of this process can be improved to save muscle proteins and other tissues.

Hormonal adaptations

- **Increase in growth hormone (GH):** GH secretion can increase significantly, promoting lipolysis (the breakdown of fat) and the preservation of muscle and bone mass. GH also helps support cell repair and renewal.
- **Increased BDNF.** Brain-derived neurotrophic factor (BDNF) may also be elevated, which supports neurogenesis and brain plasticity, and could improve cognitive function. BDNF plays a crucial role in protecting against neuronal stress and promoting a healthy nervous system.
- **Changes in insulin and leptin levels.** Reducing insulin levels improves insulin sensitivity, while altering leptin levels can affect the sensation of hunger and potentially reduce appetite.

Autophagy

- **Activation of autophagy.** Autophagy is intensified. This process cleans cells of damaged components and helps prevent age-related diseases and cell dysfunction.

Water conservation and electrolyte adjustments

- **Hydration management.** The body adjusts its water conservation mechanisms to minimise water loss, notably by reducing urine production. Electrolyte management becomes crucial to prevent imbalances, which can be critical after prolonged dry fasting.

2. Effects on overall health

In summary, after 72 hours of dry fasting, the body has activated advanced mechanisms to manage the prolonged absence of food and water intake. These adaptations support survival and homeostasis. It is crucial to stress that the phenomena described during a dry fast lasting more than three days can vary considerably depending on a number of individual factors. Personal experience of fasting, particularly dry fasting training, plays an important role in how the body reacts to this prolonged deprivation of food and water. Here are some key factors that can influence physiological and metabolic responses to dry fasting:

Dry fasting training

- Individuals accustomed to dry fasting may experience faster and more effective adaptations, with potentially fewer negative side effects, thanks to better hormonal and metabolic regulation prepared by previous dry fasting experiences.

Physical activity

- Physical activity during fasting influences the rate at which energy reserves are consumed and can affect the production of hormones such as growth hormone and BDNF. Light to moderate activity can promote the beneficial effects of dry fasting, whereas intense activity without adequate fluid intake can increase the risk of dehydration and exhaustion. It is therefore important not to engage in just any physical activity during a dry fast. We recommend caution during a dry fasting cure, as you mustn't spend your energy reserves indiscriminately.

Weight and Body Composition

- A person's initial body composition and weight determine the energy reserves available, such as glycogen and fat, which can affect how long the body can function effectively in a state of dry fasting.

Mental and Psychological State

- Mental resilience and attitude to fasting can influence the overall experience, including the ability to manage hunger and thirst, stress and mood changes. A positive and prepared state of mind can improve fasting tolerance and minimise perceived stress and go further in dry fasting.

Degree of intoxication

- The level of accumulated toxins in the body can affect detoxification processes during dry fasting. Individuals with a higher degree of intoxication may experience more intense detoxification symptoms but may also derive significant benefits from autophagy and accelerated cellular cleansing processes.

These individual variations underline the importance of a personalised, holistic approach to dry fasting, taking into account each person's unique circumstances and health conditions, before undertaking dry fasting, especially for a prolonged duration of more than three days.

CHAPTER 9

Why is dry fasting necessary in life?

It is often said that our body is a unique biological machine, capable of constantly regenerating and renewing itself without doing anything. While there is some truth in this assertion, it omits a crucial element: the limits of this self-regeneration in the face of modern challenges.

Our bodies have incredible capacities for adaptation and self-regeneration. Cells and cellular systems can identify and replace worn or pathologically modified biological structures. This self-regulatory mechanism is crucial to maintaining our health.

1. Why is dry fasting essential?

1. **The limits of self-regeneration.** In an ideal world, these mechanisms would function flawlessly. But why then do we grow old, fall ill and eventually die? The answer is that our modern environment is putting these adaptive capacities to the test, and they have largely been exceeded. Malnutrition, stress, pollution and modern toxins reduce the effectiveness of self-regeneration.
2. **Impact of modern toxins**. The exotoxins and endotoxins accumulated in our bodies reduce our capacity to adapt and self-regulate, even in good health. Vital energy is

wasted neutralising these poisons, reducing the body's ability to renew itself.

2. The crucial role of Dry Fasting

- **Stimulation of self-regeneration.** Dry fasting promotes detoxification and bacterial and viral infections, stimulating internal healing reserves and supporting self-renewal systems.
- **Increased renewal and rejuvenation.** Practical experience shows that renewal and rejuvenation of the body are greatly enhanced during dry fasting. By stopping external cell feeding for a strictly calculated period, it becomes possible to eliminate dead cells more effectively, use up old cells, cleanse diseased tissues, and remove accumulated waste and toxins.
- **A temporary break for preventive repair.** Fasting can be seen as a temporary break, allowing preventive repair of systems and mechanisms that cannot be repaired during the often-trying pace of daily life.

Conclusion

Therapeutic fasting is not simply a tool for living an experience, losing a little weight or practising an ascetic ritual. It is a biological necessity in our modern world. It offers an opportunity to reset and reinvigorate our natural capacity for self-healing, a capacity often hampered by the constraints of our misguided lifestyles. By integrating dry fasting into our lives, we can take control of our power of renewal and live a healthier, more balanced life.

3. Dry fasting and BDNF

BDNF (Brain-Derived Neurotrophic Factor) is an essential protein in the brain, promoting the growth, development and survival of nerve cells. High levels of BDNF are associated with better cognitive function and a reduced risk of neurological disorders.

Dry fasting and even intermittent fasting have been shown to have potential positive effects on BDNF. Periods of food deprivation can induce metabolic stress, prompting the body to activate defence mechanisms, including an increase in BDNF. This response could help protect brain cells and stimulate neurogenesis, encouraging the formation of new neurons.

Neurodegenerative diseases, such as Alzheimer's, Parkinson's and multiple sclerosis, are characterised by the progressive degeneration of nerve cells. Reduced levels of BDNF have been observed in some of these conditions.

Increasing BDNF may potentially offer benefits in the context of neurodegenerative diseases due to its neuroprotective effects. It may help to stimulate the survival of neurons, promote the growth of new neurons and improve synaptic plasticity.

4. Dry fasting stimulates the stem cells that repair us

Dry fasting not only activates autophagy, but also a process of spontaneous generation and rejuvenation within your cells by stem cells. Understanding the complex mechanism of dry fasting and its impact on autophagy reveals a transformative pathway to cell renewal.

In our bodies, many of us harbour a multitude of sick and toxic cells. Dry fasting triggers autophagy, as we point out several times in this book, a process of cellular recycling that involves sacrificing sick and dying cells. This detoxification process is crucial. By eliminating these toxic cells, you create an environment conducive to the regeneration of stem cells. The rejection of cellular debris frees up space for healthy cells to flourish, contributing to an overall rejuvenation of your biological system.

Stem cells are the unsung heroes within our bodies, playing an essential role in our immune system, recovery, growth and other vital functions. The therapeutic potential of stem cells is underlined by the boom in the stem cell treatment industry, estimated to be worth several trillion dollars. From the treatment of burn victims to the fight against cancer, neurological disorders and much more, the versatility of stem cells in medical applications is vast and constantly expanding.

Naturally, our bodies produce stem cells, with a significant peak during childhood and adolescence. However, as the inevitable process of ageing takes place, stem cell production declines. Herein lies the profound connection between dry fasting and immune health. By adopting a carefully executed dry fasting routine, one day a week or one or two weeks a year, you allow your body to increase its natural production of stem cells.

The revitalising effects of dry fasting on stem cell regeneration offer immense promise for boosting the immune system. By allowing your body to produce more stem cells, you create a reservoir of defence and recovery mechanisms, contributing to a healthier, more resilient immune system. In short, dry fasting, when undertaken with precision, offers a holistic approach to boosting your body's innate ability to regenerate and thrive, paving the way for improved well-being.

During dry fasting, the body enters a special metabolic state of protection and stimulation. This period of deprivation encourages the body to mobilise its energy reserves. More specifically, fasting, and dry fasting in particular, has the ability to stimulate the production of stem cells. Stem cells play a central role in tissue regeneration, repairing damage and strengthening the immune system. Fasting creates an environment conducive to the release of growth factors that promote the proliferation and differentiation of stem cells.

Fasting triggers beneficial adaptive responses, in particular the stimulation of stem cell reservoirs in various tissues. This practice is proving to be a valuable ally in promoting cell regeneration and stimulating stem cells.

5. Dry fasting and pathologies

Let's call an illness or pathology a temporary state and an effort that the body makes to re-establish an inner balance, giving the body the signal that changes need to be initiated. The body moves from its stable, balanced state to another, uncharacteristically diseased state. A body that has become unbalanced as a result of an illness makes an effort (and therefore expends vitality and energy) to return to its initial healthy state. An acute illness is a period during which the body tries to restore its previous state by activating vital forces and wasting energy. Signs of acute illness such as fever, loss of appetite and fatigue indicate the following. A fever means that the vital force has been activated and that the body is ridding itself of the cause of the illness by sweating.

Loss of appetite indicates that the vital force is preserved because it is no longer spent on digestion. Fatigue indicates that the vital force is preserved because it is no longer spent on physical activities and the body's secondary activities. People recover completely from an acute condition if they have an adequate reserve of vital force and preserve it by refusing to eat food and by remaining at rest. Medicines and antipyretics are not recommended. On the contrary, they stop, suppress and damage the body's natural defence process. The real doctors of antiquity and modern medicine have done their utmost to facilitate this innate process, which is written into our genes.

There is no point in always trying to treat everything with a long dry fast. It is often sufficient to skip a few meals at the start of the illness to avoid a serious condition. If the functional disorders are still insignificant, as indicated by a loaded tongue, headaches, a feeling of general malaise and other equally minor symptoms, short-term fasting is sufficient for the body to eliminate the intoxication before developing a serious form.

If a person fasts in a calm environment at the first signs of illness, acute illness will be mild and short-lived in most cases. A patient experiences less discomfort, less pain, no fever, less weight loss, few complications following illness, and the duration is much shorter than in patients who continue to eat when they are ill. There is only one conclusion to be drawn: as soon as you feel the symptoms of an acute condition, such as loss of appetite and high fever, start dry fasting immediately and you will recover quickly and without complications.

6. Dry fasting and hormesis

Research into health and well-being has revealed increasing evidence in favour of the idea that moderate stress can have beneficial effects on the human body. One concept that fits perfectly with this perspective is the 'law of hormesis', a biological principle according to which small amounts of stress can stimulate favourable adaptive responses.

Dry fasting, which consists of abstaining from consuming both food and liquids, has gained popularity in recent years as a method with potential health benefits. This chapter explores the relationship between the law of hormesis and dry fasting, highlighting the underlying biological mechanisms and the implications for human health.

- **The law of hormesis and its applications**

The law of hormesis is based on the principle that mild but repeated stresses can trigger adaptive responses that strengthen the body's resilience. These adaptive responses can include improvements in the regulation of oxidative stress, the inflammatory response and cellular repair. Examples of hormetic stress include moderate physical exercise, exposure to extreme temperatures and, of course, dry fasting.

- **Dry fasting and hormonal stress**

Dry fasting creates physiological stress, prompting the body to adapt in order to maintain its homeostasis. During dry fasting, the body mobilises its energy reserves, activates cellular cleansing mechanisms such as autophagy and optimises the use of nutrients. These adaptive responses can be seen as manifestations of the law of hormesis, in which stress induces positive changes in cellular functioning.

- **Biological mechanisms of dry fasting**

Several biological mechanisms are activated during dry fasting, contributing to its beneficial effects. Autophagy is stimulated to maintain cell integrity. In addition, dry fasting can induce an improvement in insulin sensitivity, promoting more efficient glucose management.

- **Implications for human health**

Although further research is needed to fully understand the long-term effects of dry fasting on human health, preliminary studies suggest potential benefits. These include weight management, improved metabolic health and even positive effects on longevity. However, it is essential to note that dry fasting is not suitable for everyone, and its application should be carried out with caution, under the supervision of a health professional.

The law of hormesis thus offers an intriguing insight into how moderate stresses can lead to beneficial adaptations in the human body. Dry fasting, as a potential hormetic stress, opens up exciting avenues for future research into the regulation of metabolism and overall health. Dry fasting remains the most powerful and effective hormone therapy known to date.

CHAPTER 10

Studies on dry fasting

1. The Russian patent for Leonid Ščennikov's health rehabilitation system

In the Russian Federation, Dr Ščennikov was the first to obtain a patent for an invention considered almost unscientific at the time. Patent no. 2028160 for invention in 1993: "*A method of re-educating the body*" (Technique of abstinence from water and food to cure oneself).

- **The aim of the study:**

To increase the therapeutic effect of therapeutic fasting, by creating a complete and highly effective methodology for combating various diseases for use in clinical and private conditions.

- **Dry fasting method:**

Detoxify the body of these wastes, restore the body's immunological status, increase the body's resistance to external influences (hormesis law), prevent and eliminate physical and psychological disorders of the human body.

The method, hereinafter referred to *as the "abstinence cure method", was* officially tested in 1992 on a group of 19 people, including one member of the expert commission, in accordance with an agreement signed with the Ivanovo Institute of Public Medicine (IGMI), the Research and Production Enterprise for Environmental Medicines, Oncological Protection and the Ivanov Gastroenterological Sanatorium in Russia.

The group included people aged between 20 and 63 suffering from hypertension, osteochondrosis, cardiovascular disease, lung cancer, bronchial asthma, kidney stones, digestive disorders, gastric ulcers, varicose veins, metabolic disorders, chronic ENT disorders, various autoimmune diseases and uterine fibroids.

Approval took place under sanatorium conditions and was overseen by a committee of competent experts made up of:

- Chernobrovy V.F. – Vice-rector for medical work at the IGMI, head of the infectious diseases department, Professor;
  Bobkov V.A. – Head of the Department of Internal Medicine, Professor;
  Poltyrev V.S. – Head of the Department of Internal Medicine, Faculty of Medicine, Professor
- Nikolayenkov Yu.V. – Vice-Rector for Academic Affairs, IGMI, Head of the Department of Pathophysiology, Professor;
- Citizen L.S. – Head of the Department of Normal Physiology, Professor;
- Slobodin V.B. – Head of the Biochemistry Department, Professor.

Experimental testing of L. A. Chennikov's abstinence cure method was accompanied by in-depth clinical evaluation and monitoring of biochemical, immunological and physiological parameters (blood tests). The dynamics of blood, urine, blood pressure and changes in body weight were taken into account by the committee of experts who examined the clinical, laboratory and functional documentation for the clinical trials of the dry fasting method. The dynamics of the changes in indicators, the phases of resistance, and the types and nature of the cleansing of the body of toxins were also taken into account.

L.A. Chennikov presented a report on the *"Cure by abstinence from water and solids"* method. The results of the clinical experiment carried out to evaluate this method were presented by IGMI associate professor E. V. Putintsev, who was one of the participants in the experiment. Clinical, laboratory and functional studies, together with a survey of patients who had undergone a two-week course of dry fasting (including two days of preparation and three days of discharge), led to the following conclusions:

1. From 12.10 to 26.10.92, Associate Professor E.V. Putintsev attended a Healing Abstinence course using the method of L.A. Chennikov. The group of participants consisted of 20 people and the head of a scientific experiment, the chief physician, V. Bunin, head of the children's gastro-enterological sanatorium in Ivanovo.
2. The committee of experts confirms the reliability of all the clinical, laboratory and functional documentation of the "Healing Abstinence" clinical trial.
3. The committee of experts confirms all the results of the scientific experiment *"Healing: abstinence from water and solids"*, which refer to the dynamics of clinical symptoms, the types and nature of the symptoms of cleansing the body of toxins and diseased tissues, the modification of phases of resistance, the dynamics of energy and vascular parameters.
4. The committee of experts confirmed the positive results reported in 18 out of 20 patients, with an improvement in blood counts.
5. The expert commission recommends the use of the method of *"healing by abstinence from water and solids" for* therapeutic purposes in a wide range of pathologies.
6. Assessment of the 96% reliability of the dry fasting method for all pathologies combined.

Comment on this study.

Dr Leonid Schenikov's innovative approach to health rehabilitation is fascinating, marked by the award of a Russian patent for his system of body re-education based on a method of abstinence from food and water. This was a significant achievement at a time when such methods were generally regarded as unscientific.

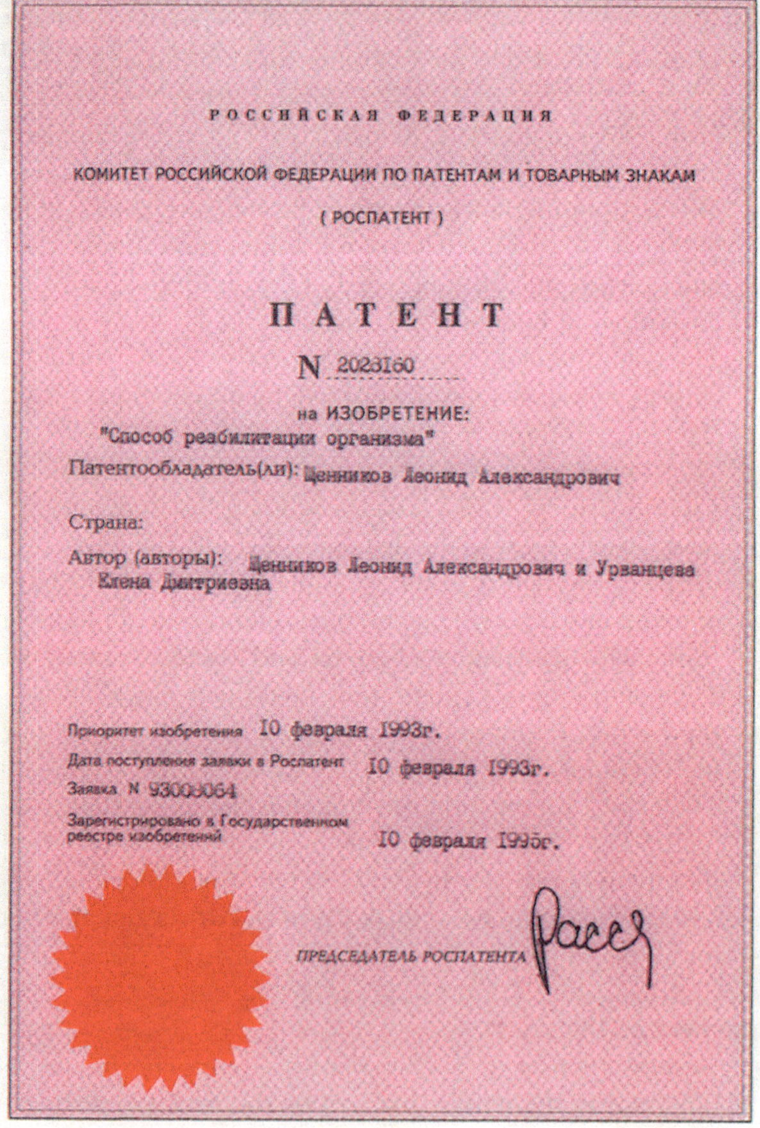

РОССИЙСКАЯ ФЕДЕРАЦИЯ

КОМИТЕТ РОССИЙСКОЙ ФЕДЕРАЦИИ ПО ПАТЕНТАМ И ТОВАРНЫМ ЗНАКАМ

(РОСПАТЕНТ)

ПАТЕНТ

N 2023160

на ИЗОБРЕТЕНИЕ:
"Способ реабилитации организма"

Патентообладатель(ли): Щенников Леонид Александрович

Страна:

Автор (авторы): Щенников Леонид Александрович и Урванцева Елена Дмитриевна

Приоритет изобретения 10 февраля 1993г.

Дата поступления заявки в Роспатент 10 февраля 1993г.

Заявка N 93006064

Зарегистрировано в Государственном реестре изобретений 10 февраля 1995г.

ПРЕДСЕДАТЕЛЬ РОСПАТЕНТА

The aim of the study, focused on improving the therapeutic effect of fasting, reveals a desire to explore holistic approaches to combating various diseases. The entire methodology focuses on detoxifying the body, restoring immunological status and increasing the body's resistance to external influences, following the law of hormesis.

The results of the clinical trial demonstrate a number of positive points. The abstinence-based cure method proved to be safe, leading to significant weight loss and a marked improvement in renal function, with a 167% increase in mean creatinine clearance.

The conclusions of the expert commission, made up of renowned medical professionals, confirm the reliability of the clinical results. The positive results in 18 out of 20 patients, with an improvement in blood counts, together with the recommendation to use this method for a wide range of pathologies, attest to the perceived efficacy of the dry fasting method and open up broad therapeutic prospects for virtually all pathologies.

2. Study on short dry fasts during Ramadan

The study entitled "Metabolic Response to Daytime Dry Fasting in Bahá'í Volunteers," published on PubMed (https://pubmed.ncbi.nlm.nih.gov/35011024/, explores the effects of daytime dry fasting, observed during the Ramadan fast, a religious practice involving abstention from food and drink from sunrise to sunset for 19 days in March. Carried out on 11 healthy men, the study measures anthropometric parameters, metabolic markers in venous blood, and pre- and postprandial energy metabolism at systemic and tissue level.

1. **Reduction in anthropometric parameters**: During dry fasting, a reduction in body weight, body mass index (BMI), body fat and blood glucose was observed.

2. **Effects on energy metabolism:** A reduction in the postprandial increase in energy expenditure and a tendency towards a reduction in diet-induced thermogenesis were observed during fasting.

3. **Tissue changes:**
   - In adipose tissue, perfusion, glucose supply and lipolysis increased.
   - In skeletal muscle, tissue perfusion did not change. Glucose supply and lipolysis decreased, while glucose oxidation increased, suggesting an improvement in insulin sensitivity.

4. **Conclusion:** The results suggest that fasting may be a promising approach to weight loss, improving metabolism and health.

Comment: This study offers interesting insights into the effects of daytime dry fasting, particularly in the context of religious fasting. The observations of reductions in body weight, BMI and blood glucose, associated with metabolic changes at the tissue level, suggest potential health benefits. However, it is crucial to note that these results are specific to Bahá'í fasting and that other forms of dry fasting may have different effects. Furthermore, the finding that, outside the context of religious fasting, skipping an evening meal may be advisable due to an apparent reduction in evening metabolism, offers an interesting perspective for dietary practices. However, further research is needed to confirm these observations and fully understand the implications for general health.

3. Physiology of dry fasting: responses to hypovolaemia and hypertonicity

Ioannis-Eleemon Papagiannopoulos, Maria Papagiannopoulou, Vassilis Sideris **https://pubmed.ncbi.nlm.nih.gov/31958788/**

Aim of the study: The aim of this study, conducted in 2020, was to gain a deeper understanding of the physiology of dry fasting (DF).

Methodology: Ten participants underwent dry fasting for five days, and various parameters were measured daily, covering hormonal, metabolic and physiological aspects.

- **Main results:**

1. **Increase in certain parameters:**
   - Hormones such as ADH, ACTH, cortisol, CRP, renin, angiotensin II and aldosterone increased.
   - Increase in total antioxidant capacity (TAC), uric acid, albumin, erythrocytes, haematocrit and noradrenalin.
   - Urine osmolality and CRP also increased.

2. **Reduction in certain parameters**:
   - Waist circumference and body weight were reduced.
   - Decrease in erythropoietin, adrenaline and sodium (Na+).
   - Vitamin C decreased, with a half-life of 4.8 ± 0.7 days.

3. **Analysis of weight loss components:**
   - The components lost were mainly urine, insensible water loss, faeces and respiratory gases.

4. **Conclusion:** The study suggests mechanisms underlying the compensation of hypertonicity and hypovolaemia during dry fasting. Dry fasting demonstrated short-term effects, including antioxidant, anti-ischaemic, immunostimulant, anti-oedematous and anti-inflammatory effects. The results suggest that dry fasting could influence new concepts for the treatment of oedema, obesity and inflammatory and ischaemic diseases.

Commentary:

This study sheds interesting light on the physiological responses to dry fasting. The hormonal and metabolic changes and physiological adjustments observed highlight the significant impact of dry fasting on the body. The antioxidant, anti-inflammatory and immunostimulant effects suggest potential implications for the management of various health problems. However, it is important to note that this study is limited by its small sample size and short duration. Further research, including longer-term studies on larger populations, is needed to confirm and extend these observations and to explore the potential benefits of longer dry fasts, which could be even more beneficial.

4. Safety of dry fasting and improvement in certain health parameters.

2013 German scientific study

Anthropometric, haemodynamic, metabolic and renal responses during five days of food and water deprivation.

Ioannis A. Papagiannopoulos 1, Vassilis I. Sidéris , Michael Boschmann , Olga S. Koutsoni , Eleni N. Dotsika

PMID: 24434757 https://pubmed.ncbi.nlm.nih.gov/24434757/

Although there is considerable research into fasting and water restriction, little is known about the impact of food and water deprivation (dry fasting) on body circumferences and vital parameters.

Method: During five days of dry fasting in ten healthy adults, haemodynamic, metabolic and renal parameters, such as weight, five circumferences at the neck, waist, hip, underarm chest, nipple chest and one new oblique hip circumference, were measured daily. For each circumference, new quotients of daily decrease in circumference in relation to weight were calculated. All the parameters used quantified and monitored compliance and effectiveness of the method by dieters.

Results: Blood pressure, heart rate, haemoglobin oxygen saturation, glucose, K(+), Na(+), Cl(-), urea, creatinine and serum osmolality were stable. Mean creatinine clearance increased by up to 167%. The mean daily weight loss (1390 ± 60 g) demonstrated the efficacy of dry fasting in weight reduction. The daily decrease in all measured circumferences and the corresponding circumference-weight decrease quotient values reflected a considerable decrease in the volume of all body parts measured per day and kg of weight loss during dry fasting.

Conclusion: The five-day dry fasting intervention in ten healthy adults proved safe, reduced weight and all measured circumferences, and significantly improved renal function.

Commentary:

This study on the impact of food and water deprivation for five days in ten healthy adults offers interesting insights into the body's physiological responses and affords a wide avenue of exploration into the management of numerous pathologies. However, the study did not go far enough, as the second acidosis crisis occurred on Day 9, and the effects would have been even greater. The results indicate stability in several vital parameters such as blood pressure, heart rate and haemoglobin oxygen saturation, suggesting a certain resilience of the cardiovascular and respiratory systems during a dry fast of just five days. A striking feature of the study was the significant increase in mean creatinine clearance of up to 167%, suggesting a marked improvement in renal function. This observation could be of particular interest in understanding the effects of dry fasting on the body's purification systems, although further studies are needed to investigate this further. It also opens up observations on the possible cure of all kidney diseases.

The effectiveness of dry fasting in reducing weight was also demonstrated, with a mean daily weight reduction of 1390 ± 60 g. This raises questions about the mechanisms underlying this weight loss, including the relative contribution of water loss, mobilisation of glycogen reserves and lipolysis. Another perspective could be to further explore compliance and tolerance of the method, given that dry fasting can be considered a radical approach and requires professional monitoring to ensure the safety and well-being of the dry faster. In summary, this study suggests that dry fasting for five days in healthy adults is safe, induces significant weight loss, and has positive effects on renal function. However, further research is needed to fully understand the underlying mechanisms and to assess the long-term implications of this method on overall health. Furthermore, we do not know under what conditions the study took place, as the authors of the study are not specialists in dry fasting. Professional guidance and the location of the fast may further improve the results of the study.

5. Intermittent fasting during Ramadan

Attenuation of pro-inflammatory cytokines and immune cells in healthy subjects

Mo'ez Al-Islam E Faris, Safia Kacimi, Ref'at A Al-Kurd, Mohammad A Fararjeh, Yasser K Bustanji, Mohammad K Mohammad, Mohammad L Salem (2012)

https://pubmed.ncbi.nlm.nih.gov/23244540/

Summary: Intermittent fasting and caloric restriction have been shown to prolong life expectancy and reduce inflammation and cancer in animal models. We hypothesised that prolonged intermittent fasting during the month of Ramadan (RIF) could have a positive impact on the inflammatory state. To investigate this hypothesis, a cross-sectional study was designed to examine the impact of RIF on selected inflammatory cytokines and immune biomarkers in healthy subjects. Fifty healthy volunteers (21 men and 29 women) practising the Ramadan fast were recruited for the study of circulating pro-inflammatory cytokines, immune cells (total leukocytes, monocytes, granulocytes and lymphocytes), as well as anthropometric and dietary assessments. Investigations were carried out one week before the Ramadan fast, at the end of the third week of Ramadan and one month after the end of Ramadan. Pro-inflammatory cytokines and tumour necrosis factor, systolic and diastolic blood pressure, body weight and percentage body fat were significantly lower ($P < .05$) during Ramadan compared with before Ramadan or after the cessation of Ramadan fasting. Immune cells decreased significantly during Ramadan but remained within the reference ranges. These results indicate that RIF attenuates the inflammatory state of the body by suppressing the expression of pro-inflammatory cytokines and decreasing body fat and circulating leucocyte levels.

- **Dry fasting and reduced inflammation**

The link between dry fasting and reduced inflammation has also been studied. In a 2012 study published in Nutrition Research, scientists measured the pro-inflammatory cytokines of 50 healthy adults one week before Ramadan. This measurement was repeated during the third week and one month after they practised dry fasting during Ramadan.

Participants' levels of pro-inflammatory cytokines were lowest during the third week of dry fasting. This suggests a reduction in inflammation during fasting, which may improve the immune system. However, it is important to note that fasting during Ramadan is not continuous and water is allowed at certain times.

The link between dry fasting and improved immune function requires further research.

- **Fasting in general reduces inflammation and dry fasting even more so**

Inflammation is a natural reaction by the body in response to aggression. However, when this reaction becomes excessive or inappropriate, it can contribute to the development of pathological phenomena. A number of regulatory pathways that directly or indirectly influence the inflammatory response are currently being studied. Among these, the regulatory pathways of cellular metabolism appear to play an increasingly obvious role in regulating the inflammatory status of various immune cells. Immunometabolism, a growing field of research, could help to elucidate the pathophysiological mechanisms underlying many diseases.

With the widespread adoption of Western dietary habits and increased consumption of high-energy foods, excess caloric intake is frequently observed worldwide. This excess is associated with the establishment of a chronic systemic inflammatory state, contributing to the development of inflammatory metabolic diseases such as type 2 diabetes and atherosclerosis. Excess calorie intake is also implicated in the development of inflammatory and autoimmune diseases. On the other hand, research has shown that fasting or low-calorie diets can have a protective effect against these diseases. Clinical studies on intermittent fasting (less than 24 hours) have revealed a reduction in levels of pro-inflammatory cytokines. However, the precise mechanisms by which a reduction in calorie intake modulates systemic inflammation are still poorly understood.

- **The number of circulating pro-inflammatory monocytes decreases during a short fast.**

We can examine the impact of fasting on immune cell homeostasis, focusing particularly on monocytes. These cells selectively target inflammatory sites and play an essential role in initiating and maintaining inflammation by secreting pro-inflammatory cytokines. At tissue level, monocytes differentiate into macrophages, which also produce numerous inflammatory mediators.

In healthy subjects, the researchers observed a reduction in blood monocytes after a 19-hour fast, although their level remained within physiological limits. Similar experiments conducted on mice revealed that a short four-hour fast, equivalent to nocturnal fasting in humans, also led to a reduction in the level of pro-inflammatory monocytes.

In conclusion, after a short fast, the researchers observed that the altered expression profile of more than 2,700 genes within monocytes was responsible for a slowdown in their energy metabolism, as evidenced by the simultaneous reduction in their oxygen consumption and extracellular acidification. Given that the cytoskeletal rearrangements required for migration represent one of the most energy-intensive cellular processes, monocytes persist away from the bloodstream after fasting, thereby ceasing to exert their systemic pro-inflammatory action.

Fasting reduces the symptoms of chronic inflammatory disease without compromising the acute anti-infectious inflammatory response. Given that calorie restriction has been associated with protection against chronic inflammatory and autoimmune diseases, the researchers examined the effect of intermittent fasting in mice suffering from autoimmune encephalomyelitis, an experimental model of multiple sclerosis in which pro-inflammatory monocytes are known to be involved. They demonstrated that fasting induced an improvement in symptoms associated with a reduction in the number of pro-inflammatory monocytes infiltrating the spinal cord. These monocytes also showed an alteration in their pro-inflammatory transcriptome signature.

In addition, the results of this study, which showed a reduction in the peripheral mobilisation of pro-inflammatory monocytes, led the researchers to ask whether fasting altered the development of acute inflammatory reactions, which are essential for combating infection by pathogenic agents. In contrast to prolonged food deprivation (more than 48 hours), they showed that short fasting did not impair the antimicrobial response of mice infected with the bacterium Listeria monocytogenes, particularly in terms of monocyte recruitment at the infection site.

6. Dry fasting: an ally against muscle loss and an effective fat burner

For thousands of years, fasting has been an integral part of human nature, whether involuntary due to food shortages, or voluntary for cultural and religious reasons. Our ancestors survived thanks to an efficient system for storing and recovering energy in the form of body fat. With modern food abundance, many cultures and religions have incorporated voluntary fasting as a purification and regeneration procedure.

Impact of Fasting on Muscle Mass

Historical experience and recent clinical evidence show that fasting, whether short- or long-term, does not cause significant muscle loss. On the contrary, it appears to preserve and even improve muscle mass under certain conditions.

GENESIS study

The GENESIS study explored the effects of a 12-day fasting period on various bodily functions, including muscle metabolism. The results indicated that fasting could lead to a temporary reduction in organ size and muscle mass. However, after refeeding, there was an acceleration of protein turnover and resynthesis, suggesting rejuvenation and preservation of lean tissue after fasting.

Hormonal response

During fasting, the body increases production of counter-regulatory hormones such as growth hormone (HGH), adrenaline, noradrenaline and cortisol. HGH, in particular, helps to preserve muscle mass by promoting protein synthesis during refeeding. This hormonal response ensures that the body maintains muscle mass during periods of fasting.

Mechanisms of Muscle Preservation

Dr Jason Fung, a world specialist in water fasting, points out that during fasting, the body prioritises the preservation of muscle tissue by using fat reserves for energy. Protein catabolism (breakdown) mainly targets proteins with high turnover rates, such as those in the skin and intestinal mucosa, rather than muscle proteins. This selective breakdown of proteins helps to preserve muscle mass during prolonged fasting.

Re-feeding phase

The refeeding phase is crucial for maintaining muscle mass. When fasting ends and normal eating resumes, the body uses the available nutrients to rebuild and repair muscle tissue more effectively, thanks to elevated levels of growth hormone and insulin. This process not only restores, but can also improve muscle quality and function.

The Body's Metabolic Priorities During Fasting

During fasting, the body's priority is to maintain a sufficient level of glucose for brain function. The body switches to fat oxidation and ketone utilisation, with a significant reduction in muscle protein breakdown. Rapidly renewing proteins, such as those found in the skin and intestinal mucosa, are used preferentially, contributing to the anti-inflammatory effect observed clinically. Muscle cells, which are less frequently renewed, are spared.

The proportion of energy from protein is lower in obese subjects than in lean subjects, demonstrating that the body uses more fat when it is available. During a very prolonged 15-day water fast, obese subjects burn less protein than lean subjects.

Therapeutic dry fasting

Dry fasting preserves muscle even more and accelerates fat loss three times more than a water fast. Although research into dry fasting is limited, certain studies and observations provide clues to its effects.

Preservation of Muscles

Increase in Growth Hormone (HGH)

Fasting, including dry fasting, can lead to a significant increase in the secretion of human growth hormone (HGH). This hormone is known for its effects on preserving muscle mass. For example, one study showed that even a 24-hour fast can double or triple HGH secretion, and in the case of dry fasting, this increase can be even more pronounced. Stem cells are also increased as soon as food is resumed, further aiding the synthesis of new proteins.

Fat metabolism

Dry fasting leads to a rapid transition from carbohydrate to fat metabolism. During this period, the body mainly uses fat reserves to produce energy, which helps preserve muscle mass. Fat metabolism becomes the main source of energy, reducing the need to break down muscle proteins.

Studies on Ramadan fasting

Research into the Ramadan fast, which involves abstinence from food and water from sunrise to sunset, shows that this type of fast can help reduce body fat and improve various health indicators such as cholesterol and blood glucose levels.

A recent study of a five-day dry fast showed significant weight loss, much of which is attributed to the loss of body fat. However, it is important to note that some of this weight loss is due to water loss.

Although dry fasting appears to have beneficial effects on muscle mass preservation and fat utilisation, the available scientific data remains limited and more research is needed to fully understand these effects.

Conclusion

Fasting, whether intermittent, prolonged or dry, preserves lean tissue better than traditional weight loss methods, but support from a health professional specialising in dry fasting is necessary. The hormonal and metabolic adaptations during dry fasting, including the increase in growth hormone and counter-regulatory hormones, show that the human body is well equipped to manage periods of fasting without significant muscle loss.

Ultimately, studies and expert opinion suggest that prolonged fasting, followed by adequate refeeding, can preserve and even potentially improve muscle mass and function, challenging the common belief that fasting leads to muscle loss.

https://pubmed.ncbi.nlm.nih.gov/10837292/
https://pubmed.ncbi.nlm.nih.gov/3127426/
https://hackfasting.com/dry-fasting-benefits/does-dry-fasting-cause-muscle-loss/
https://www.dietdoctor.com/does-fasting-burn-muscle
https://www.frontiersin.org/articles/10.3389/fnut.2022.951000/full
https://www.bcm.edu/news/dawn-to-dusk-dry-fasting-leads-to-health-benefits-in-the-study-of-immune-cells

CHAPTER 11

Physical preparation for dry fasting

1. The dietary organisation chart for good preparation for dry fasting

- **Preparation by Michel Deladoey**

The points explained here are for guidance only and are not compulsory, except perhaps in the last week, when you should avoid meat, dairy products and sweets of all kinds, while favouring cooked and raw vegetables. The following information is just a suggestion. Do what you feel like doing and what is possible for you, without complicating your life or stressing yourself unnecessarily.

Three proposals for food descent

1.1 The advantages of the ketogenic diet in preparing for a dry fast

Therapeutic dry fasting has gained in popularity in recent years due to its potential health benefits, which are superior to any other type of fasting. Combined with the ketogenic diet, dry fasting can be optimised to maximise its therapeutic benefits. We will explore in detail the benefits of the ketogenic diet as a preparation for therapeutic dry fasting for those who want it.

The ketogenic diet, often referred to as keto, is an eating plan that focuses on high fat consumption, moderate protein and low carbohydrate content. The main aim is to induce a metabolic state called ketosis, in which the body burns fat to produce energy instead of glucose from carbohydrates.

- **Advantage 1: Smooth transition to ketosis**

By adopting the ketogenic diet before starting a dry fast, the body gradually enters a state of ketosis. This smooth transition allows the metabolism to adjust to using ketones as the main source of energy. This can reduce initial fasting symptoms such as fatigue and headaches, making the dry fasting process easier.

- **Advantage 2: Stabilisation of blood sugar levels**

The ketogenic diet helps to stabilise blood sugar levels by limiting carbohydrate consumption. Stable blood sugar levels are essential to prepare the body for dry fasting, as they help to avoid dramatic insulin fluctuations. Glycaemic stability can reduce feelings of hunger and energy fluctuations during dry fasting.

- **Benefit 3: Increased Stress Resistance**

The ketosis induced by the ketogenic diet has demonstrated positive effects on resistance to cellular stress. By optimising the capacity of cells to use ketones as a source of energy, the ketogenic diet can potentially reduce cellular damage during dry fasting. This could have important implications for the prevention of oxidative stress associated with fasting.

- **Advantage 4: Preservation of muscle mass**

One of the common concerns during fasting is the loss of muscle mass. The ketogenic diet, by providing adequate protein and stimulating the production of ketones, may play a role in preserving muscle mass during dry fasting. This may be particularly beneficial for those seeking to maintain their muscular health during the fasting period.

In conclusion, the ketogenic diet can provide a solid basis for preparing the body for therapeutic dry fasting. By exploiting the benefits of ketosis, blood sugar stabilisation and muscle preservation, this combined approach could improve the efficacy and tolerance of dry fasting.

1.2 The advantages of the dissociated diet in preparation for dry fasting

The importance of separating carbohydrates and proteins in preparation for dry fasting

The dissociated diet, often referred to as the Hay dissociated diet, is distinguished by its fundamental principle of rigorous separation of carbohydrates and proteins during meals. This dietary model proposes that these two nutritional groups should not be consumed simultaneously, thus highlighting the importance of specific dissociation to optimise preparation for therapeutic dry fasting. In this chapter, we will explore the advantages of specifically dissociating carbohydrates from proteins, with an emphasis on eating one low-carbohydrate meal a day. The dissociated diet advocates a strict dissociation between carbohydrates and proteins in order to promote better digestion and maximise health benefits.

- **Advantage 1: Optimisation of digestion by dissociation of nutrients**

The dissociation of carbohydrates and proteins in the dissociated diet optimises digestion by avoiding the simultaneous consumption of these two food groups. By concentrating on this separation, the diet facilitates the breakdown of nutrients more efficiently, thereby reducing stress on the digestive system. This practice is crucial in preparing the body for dry fasting by promoting simplified digestion.

- **Advantage 2: Stimulation of autophagy through carbohydrate reduction**

By dissociating carbohydrates from proteins, the diet focuses on reducing carbohydrates, which could potentially stimulate autophagy. Reducing carbohydrate intake could trigger periods of intermittent fasting, thereby promoting the autophagy process. This specific approach to dietary dissociation may amplify the benefits of autophagy, paving the way for therapeutic dry fasting.

- **Advantage 3: Managing insulin sensitivity with a low-carbohydrate meal**

A crucial aspect of the dissociated diet is the preference for one low-carb meal a day. By eliminating the consumption of carbohydrates in a daily meal, the diet promotes improved management of insulin sensitivity. This feature becomes particularly relevant in the context of dry fasting, helping to minimise fluctuations in blood sugar levels and prepare the body for a prolonged period of fasting.

In conclusion, the specific dissociation of carbohydrates and proteins, combined with a low-carbohydrate daily meal, represents a potentially effective strategy in preparation for therapeutic dry fasting. By optimising digestion, stimulating autophagy through carbohydrate reduction and improving insulin sensitivity, this approach focuses on specific benefits for a smooth transition to dry fasting.

1.3 Specific preparation for long dry fasts of up to ten days – Michel Deladoey

This should be done as soon as possible before the dry fast you are about to undertake. There are no rules; you can apply several therapies in succession or at the same time, or even juggle the different ideas for preparations suggested below. The therapy can also be highly individualised, depending on your personal characteristics. Your therapist will be able to give you the best advice on the order to follow and the supplements to combine.

1. As far as possible, start with intermittent water fasting for 16 hours. Eat your last meal at 8 pm maximum and your next meal at 12 pm the following day. If it's difficult not to eat and you're very active, just eat an avocado, vegetables and eggs (but not hard-boiled eggs). I can also recommend eating an oxidised banana for a few hours or even overnight if you tolerate it well. You can add a little ground almond or protein powder. Do not mix bananas with watery fruits such as apples or pears.

2. As soon as possible, from four months to two weeks before the long dry fasting cure, do short dry fasts of 24h or 36h each week, if you can manage it. The 24-hour dry fast is done from midday to midday. If this is too difficult psychologically, do it at least every two weeks. The more short dry fasts you do, the easier your long cure will be, with less waste and toxins to evacuate. You can also do three days of dry fasting one to three months before the cure to reassure yourself and see what is already happening. It's easier to do this over a weekend.

3. As soon as you can, cleanse yourself of general toxins with clinopitilolite active zeolite. Take one scoop twice a day before meals or between meals. Find a good quality retailer. I use Dr Niedermeier's German brand, which you can also find in France or Switzerland in pharmacies. Take zeolite for a maximum of six weeks, twice a year.

   Instead of zeolite, you can take a course of ventilated green clay such as Argiletz organic clay or Argileo, which mixes two different types of clay. Pour in one wooden teaspoon, stir and wait at least 15 minutes or, better still, overnight.

Then drink the entire glass, two hours after meals or other food supplements. For the first week, take just one teaspoon, then two. Above all, never take castor oil and clay on the same day, as you run the risk of occlusion. Duration of clay cure: three weeks.

4. If you have the time, take a course of Neem powder or capsules. I like the Organic India brand, but there are others. Take 2x 2 capsules a day for one to two months. This will already have a positive effect on your overall health and provide a complete cleansing and light detox. Neem has many benefits. Take it with meals. The dosage should be adjusted in consultation.

5. The best remedy to prepare for dry fasting is Fir resin. You can take the neem and the fir resin together, but you can also do just the neem or the resin during the day. But doing both is even better. One to three months before, start with one teaspoon of fir resin, two to three times a day, ten minutes before a meal or between meals. This can also replace coffee in the morning on an empty stomach, by adding the resin to warm water but not too hot. It will work on the pathogens that are underestimated in most people, initially draining the lymphatic system and cleansing the liver and intestines. The action of this product is to remove what is necrotic and clean the cells. On its own, it is an excellent preparation for a dry fast one to three months beforehand. This product can be taken every day to remineralise and help in all cases. It will also have a general remineralising action before the dry fast. This product will also be of interest at the end of a dry fast to remineralise and base the body, which was acidified during the cure. You can start the first week with one teaspoon to get used to it. You can choose to take this product only with the dry fast and the preparation will be excellent.

The product is explained in detail on my online shop page:
www.jeunesec.com
Video explanation on https://www.youtube.com/watch?v=_G3VZt3sg4Y&t=4s

6. Eat organic wherever possible. Avoid dairy products and gluten-based products (wheat, barley, rye, oats, quinoa, millet, buckwheat). Eliminate industrial products. Eat eggs for the last three weeks and avoid white and red meat.

7. As soon as you can and if you have time, for at least two months, do a specific drainage and regeneration of the liver with three plants. The liver is a key organ that needs to be cleansed and harmonised as much as possible, as it handles 400 functions in our body. Take one teaspoon of quantis in water, just before meals, twice a day.
Quantis 2 vials.
Turmeric, milk thistle, artichoke in equal parts. www.LPEV.fr
For Swiss callers, freephone: 0 800 56 33 82
For Belgians, freephone: 0 80071098
For French customers +33 4 70 90 61 45
If you are asked for a practitioner number: 14 90 664

8. Chew your food and eat little during the last three weeks, put your dishes on the table and don't move around, eat in a quiet place without television. Eating with chopsticks is a good way of slowing down.

9. Avoid sugar and products containing refined sugar where the packets mention fructose. Remove all industrial products, biscuits, coffee, cheese and yoghurt for the last three weeks. Eliminate alcohol. But you can consume two squares of dark chocolate for up to ten days before the dry fast.

10. Above all, don't mix starches with proteins at the same meal in the last month. For example, have a lunchtime meal of quinoa, buckwheat, rice or potatoes with raw and cooked vegetables. For dinner, eat fish, eggs, chicken or seafood with raw or cooked vegetables. Seaweed can be mixed into any meal. I recommend sea beans, dulse nori and samphire, even in jars. It's interesting from a nutritional point of view. If you have digestive problems, avoid too much raw food, which can irritate the digestive mucosa. To sum up, eat a carbohydrate meal at lunchtime and a ketogenic meal in the evening, with vegetables and proteins in the evening. But if you can, try to replace the seeds and cereals with carrots, potatoes, sweet potatoes or konjac, all of which are easier to digest. The aim is to facilitate digestion, which will help you gain as much vital energy as possible to facilitate dry fasting later on.

11. From time to time, eat only one stewed fruit as dessert, which is easier to digest after a meal.

12. Read labels and avoid food additives containing E, because even organic food contains them. Avoid fructose and all synthetic vitamins.

13. Steam your vegetables gently, using a wicker basket or a Baumstal-type vitaliser.

14. Ban the microwave oven as it can cause cancer over time. Check that the restaurants you frequent don't use them.

15. Use quality water, i.e. without chlorine. The water in Swiss towns and villages is generally chlorinated and therefore affects the digestive microbiota. You need spring water or a Berkley-type water filtration system or one with dynamisation. If you don't have any of these, use bottled water such as Mont Roucous, Montcalm or Rosée de la

reine. But you'll need to revitalise it because bottled water is dead. For bottled water, revitalise it with a drawing of a flower of life, a shape-wave device that restructures the water, Koltsov plates, or a written word (e.g. love), which you place under the bottle. Magnets can also be used. You can also revitalise the water by placing it in a glass carafe in the sun.

13. Recover as much energy as possible before the dry fast, by sleeping early if possible, no later than 10pm. Ideally, you should get nine hours' sleep.

14. In the morning, especially during the 24- or 36-hour dry fast in the preparatory phase, do ice water affusions if you like or a bucket of water over your head, with water at less than 11 degrees. If that's not possible, take a cold shower every other day, for 30 seconds to two minutes, or even longer, depending on your capabilities. You can also go to lakes or rivers. The water should be less than +11 degrees if possible. During dry fasting, always try cold water affusions. It's not an easy thing to do, but you'll reap enormous immune, circulatory and psychological benefits. If it's too difficult, forget it. Affusions are optional; your dry fasting coach will inform you about the options you can choose.

15. Put yourself psychologically in preparation mode for your dry fast and prepare for inner change. Tell your body, your cells, that after your dry fasting cure, your life, your vital force and your inner confidence will be at their highest level. Doubt and fear will no longer be part of your life. You won't be able to carry on as before. Dry fasting will give you a fresh start. Your close friends may see you as a changed person. Certain decisions may or may not be taken after this cure, which works on physical and psycho-emotional levels. You will feel a deep inner calm for some time, and it's up to you to make the most

of it so that it lasts. You can also meditate and visualise that this retreat will go wonderfully well and that you'll experience a powerful cleansing unlike anything you've ever experienced. During these preparatory meditations, you can play soft music and visualise yourself in the field of all possibilities: a new beginning in your life will take place.

16. It should be noted that a single cure will not be enough to treat all your physical problems, because dry fasting works according to the laws of priorities and fasting will work where your body needs it, whether that's resting the organs, detoxifying or working on infections. Dry fasting works with you, where your body needs it. In the case of chronic pathologies, we recommend three to four cures over one year. This is where we have had the best results. For health prevention, seven days of dry fasting per year is ideal. Don't do any medical tests immediately after the dry fast. Wait at least six weeks before doing any tests.

17. Resume physical exercise as a matter of urgency to cleanse the kidney filters, liver and intestines and increase the mitochondria in the cells, which will help you to have more energy to keep the fast dry. Do at least 3 x 45 minutes of sport a week. Create a slight shortness of breath. If you have pain, use a trampoline or go swimming in a pool or lake. If you find it difficult to move, buy some Nordic walking poles and walk fast with them. You can also invest in a Schumann plate, which activates all the body's functions and creates beneficial vibratory movements throughout the body. But this is no substitute for physical activity. So you need to get moving. If you can, always try to breathe through your nose and close your mouth. This will bring more CO_2 into your body and oxygenate it. If you can't run, take a walk every day if possible. You can also do HIT, high-intensity interval training. This will take you less than ten minutes a day. Do a short three-minute warm-up.

Climb the stairs or walk fast, then do a 30-second session at full intensity on the stairs or a steep climb. Lower and bend your knees quickly, then take 20 seconds to recover and do the exercise again for 30 seconds at full intensity. Do this for five minutes and you'll get a good result. Start gradually if you've never done any sport in your life.

18. If you have time, say four to five months, take one or two cups a day of bicarbonate of soda in hot water, one teaspoon twice a day outside meals. This will dilute the blood and prepare you well for the dry fast. You can also do this in the last month.

19. During the last 15 days, don't do any more dry fasts. If you have about two or three months to prepare, do a gradual preparation ranging from one to three days of dry fasting. If you have two months ahead of you, do 24-hour or 36-hour dry fasts in the first month, then from the fifth week onwards, do three days of dry fasting if you're motivated. Then let three weeks go by and you'll be ready in excellent conditions. If you only have two weeks left before the fast, do just one 24-hour fast, ten days before the deadline.

20. If you have serious digestive problems, follow the Fodmap diet for the last month and, if you can, drink chicken stock, which helps to heal the digestive mucosa that has become porous over the years. Check out this recipe from Dr Natacha Campbell's GAPS diet. It will reduce digestive fermentation caused by certain foods and improve certain symptoms.

21. If you want to know what type of diet you should adopt according to your genetics, there is a test called "apoe" with the e2, e3 and e4 alleles. This can be useful for finding out whether you are more fat, carbohydrate or lipid. This is a saliva test to be carried out in a laboratory.

22. Take omega 3 with EPA and DHA for energy and to thin the blood before dry fasting: one to two capsules a day with a meal. In addition, take Vigean brand walnut or rapeseed oil, at least two tablespoons a day.

23. Purge your intestines, if you wish, with magnesium sulphate before starting dry fasting. The dosage is 30g per one litre of water. Personally, I put one large tablespoon in a large glass of water, six hours after a light meal. Elimination will take place about six to eight hours later. You can drink as it can make you thirsty. Don't eat anything for at least eight hours before taking magnesium sulphate, or start dry fasting directly afterwards.

24. The ideal solution for me, however, is to purge with Pianto (vegetable concentrate) https://www.pianto.com/. It's gentle, doesn't attack the flora or mucous membranes and recharges you with minerals.
    Dilute two heaped tablespoons in 300ml of lukewarm water. Do this at least eight hours after your last very light meal. Do this three times every hour. You can also take one teaspoon every 20 minutes according to this protocol. You can also do this at any time as a purge if you feel unwell or before fasting. In total, take Pianto 18 times a day (i.e. 18 times two teaspoons in 25cl of water).
    Example:

    - From 7am to 8am every 20 minutes (7am, 7.20am, 7.40am and 8am, i.e. four doses)
    - from 10am to 11am every 20 minutes, so four doses
    - from 1pm to 2pm every 20 minutes ...
    - from 4pm to 5pm every 20 minutes ...
    - at 7pm, 1 dose
    - at 8pm, 1 dose

    In total, over the course of the day: take 18 glasses of Pianto Juice

It's best to test this purge beforehand, as it may not be right for you.

25. I also recommend eating a last meal of cooked or raw vegetables and 24 hours later, doing an enema or two enemas with lukewarm water. Buy an enema bag from a chemist. You can also purge nothing and that's fine too. However, for some people, an enema removes matter from the colon. Be really careful to eat very lightly in the last week and especially at the last meal.

26. You can also do neither an enema nor a purge, but the last meals will be very light, with vegetables and fruit in small quantities.

27. Reduce the amount of food you eat as soon as you decide to go on a dry fast. Leave the meal with a slight feeling of hunger and without digestive pain.

28. You can keep eating chicken and quail eggs and fish in small quantities for up to five days before dry fasting.

29. Be assured that dry fasting is an extraordinary way of purifying and regenerating yourself. The only enemy you will have during your cure is the fear of dying of thirst or becoming dehydrated, which is physiologically impossible. Our bodies are perfectly equipped to last a fortnight without any water intake. Some people have even gone as long as 21 days. The kidneys continue to work because our body is made up of 70% water. So calculate your weight and see how many litres of water you have available for your dry fasting cure. Ideally, it's a good idea to do seven days and even better nine days, in order to reach the second acidosis crisis, which is often very curative, but not everyone can do it. I'll discuss the number of days with you.

30. For the last three weeks, no red or white meat. Just stick to fish and eggs. Avoid all industrial and sugary products.

31. If you have a healthy diet and are not too overloaded with toxins, a short one-week preparation, with just raw and cooked vegetables in the last week and no purging or enema, is also acceptable.

32. If you wish, you can take a drift bath, which will help with general detoxification and burn some excess fat. Choose the pouches available on yokool.co.uk, add a sock and place them in the crotch area under your underwear. Use at least two pouches a day. Cold can also be useful during dry fasting.

33. The oral flora is home to numerous bacteria that can migrate throughout the body and cause all kinds of pathologies. It's always a good idea to clean your mouth with 3% or 10-volume hydrogen peroxide: one teaspoon of hydrogen peroxide to two teaspoons of water. Then spit out the mixture and rinse your mouth. Do not swallow the mixture.
    For two months, take propolis spray in your mouth, circulate the liquid, then spit it out. Do this for at least two months, once a day. You should also have your teeth cleaned every four months and floss once a day. This simple mouth cleaning alone can improve psoriasis or an autoimmune disease. You can also rinse your mouth with coconut oil for 20 minutes using a method described in a later chapter.

34. Favour the fodmaps diet before and after dry fasting if you have digestive problems. **The most interesting vegetables are those that ferment the least**:

    - aubergine
    - chard
    - head of broccoli

- carrot
- courgette
- endive
- fennel stalk
- green spring onion stalk
- cucumber
- spinach
- ginger
- lamb's lettuce
- parsley
- red pepper
- radish
- rocket
- green salad

Although I don't really recommend starches, here's a list of starches that are low in fodmaps, but don't overuse them.

- maize starch
- maize flour
- potato flour
- rice flour
- oat flakes
- polenta
- millet
- rice noodles
- gluten-free bread
- quinoa
- rice
- buckwheat flour
- sweet potato

Dairy products and derivatives low in fodmaps
Tolerance to watch out for:

- clarified butter

- camembert, low dose
- Emmental, low dose
- feta cheese
- hard cheese, low dose
- almond milk
- coconut milk (< 150 ml)
- rice milk
- lactose-free milk
- margarine
- mozzarella, low dose
- parmesan, low dose
- milk protein
- plain coconut milk yoghurt

List of fruits low in fodmap:

- pineapple
- unripe banana
- carambola
- lemon
- clementine
- durian
- cutter
- kiwi
- kumquat
- mandarin
- chestnut
- orange
- grapes
- prickly pear
- blueberry, raspberry

35. **In case of severe digestive problems or autoimmune problems.**
    Simply cut out carbohydrates or switch to the AIP diet explained below.

2. The AIP scheme

The acronym AIP stands for Auto-Immune Protocol. To make the French translation more meaningful, the term protocole AIP is used. More than a diet, the AIP protocol is a lifestyle.

Who is it for?

As its name suggests, the Autoimmune Protocol is aimed primarily at people with autoimmune diseases, chronic illnesses and severe digestive problems. Autoimmune diseases occur when the immune system is out of control. The immune cells designed to destroy pathogens begin to attack the body's own tissues. There are no doctors specialising in autoimmune diseases. Current medicine seeks to treat the affected organ, often with lifelong treatment and side effects, whereas a change in lifestyle and specific attention to the immune system can often limit the symptoms.

In IBD, the AIP protocol could help to maintain remission while limiting symptoms. A study carried out on 16 women with Hashimoto's thyroiditis showed that after ten weeks on the AIP diet, inflammation was reduced by 29% and symptoms by 68%.

In short, the AIP protocol can be used in a number of cases: autoimmune diseases, chronic inflammatory diseases and cases of intestinal hyperpermeability.

- **What does this protocol involve?**

The protocol is based on a paleo-type elimination/reintroduction diet and the introduction of highly nutritious foods (using the principle of nutritional density). The elimination phase can be gradual or overnight, depending on individual preferences. This phase is therefore divided into two stages:

- Transition, the duration of which varies according to the pace of each individual
- Maintenance, lasting from 30 to 90 days

Once ready, the reintroduction phase can begin. The protocol also involves a 'rethink' of lifestyle: sleep, stress management, physical activity and connecting with others (and I think we can also include (re)connecting with nature).

Foods to eliminate are:

- Cereals, pseudocereals and cereal-like substances containing gluten
- Dairy products
- Legumes (including soya)
- Refined oils and sugars, as well as sweeteners
- Food additives
- Nuts and seeds
- Fruit and berry-based spices
- Solanaceae (tomatoes, chillies, potatoes, aubergines, tamarillos, goji berries, etc.)
- Eggs (no more than three a week)
- Alcohol
- Coffee

These foods are likely to over-stimulate the immune system and therefore fuel inflammation. This is not a low-carb diet in the strict sense of the word, but it can be if you choose to follow it, with the advice of your doctor, dietician or specialist naturopath.

- **What can you eat during the elimination phase?**

  - Meat from grass-fed animals
  - Fish and seafood
  - Vegetables (with exceptions, see foods to avoid above)
  - Quality oils and fats (extra virgin olive oil, coconut oil, duck fat, lard, etc.)
  - Broth (vegetable, poultry, beef...)
  - Offal

- Flours not derived from cereals or nuts (coconut flour, souchet, manioc, green banana, sweet potato, etc.)
- Starch not derived from cereals or solanaceous plants (tapioca starch, arrowroot)

The aim of the protocol is therefore to restore correct immune function and optimal digestive health, to provide nutrients and to regulate hormonal functions.

✔ The benefits

The low FODMAPs diet sometimes works miracles, but it is not enough on its own. Limiting the FODMAPs in your diet and then reintroducing them without having changed your eating habits, made up your nutritional deficiencies and optimised your digestion, won't do much good and your efforts won't have the desired results. I really like the global approach proposed by this protocol. This is personally what I insist on with my patients, whether or not they are following a low FODMAP diet: we are a whole and intestinal well-being is not independent of the rest.

✘ Disadvantages

As with any elimination/reintroduction diet, it can be difficult to get started. Depending on your current diet, your eating habits will be affected to a greater or lesser extent. Implementing the protocol requires organisation. Unlike the low FODMAPs diet, there are few tools available (no application, few resources in French) and you may feel lost and alone. To maximise your chances of success, it's essential to be accompanied by a healthcare professional.

- **In a nutshell**

Studies specific to the AIP protocol are still few and far between, but the paleo diet and its positive effects on autoimmune diseases have been better documented. Thanks to its global approach, the AIP protocol seems very promising. It would help to reduce inflammation and relieve the symptoms induced by autoimmune disease. As with any therapeutic regime, support is essential to ensure that you are meeting your needs and providing you with moral and organisational support.

3. Cleaning the organs

3.1 The Essentials of Liver Cleansing for Optimal Health

Cleansing the liver is a crucial aspect of our overall well-being and is the ideal preparation for dry fasting. It is often underestimated. Think of your liver as your body's detoxification control centre. Over time, because of our modern diet and environment, it can become clogged with toxins, affecting its ability to function effectively.

Think of the liver as a powerful filter. Just like an air filter in your home, it needs regular cleaning to maintain its performance. An uncleaned liver is like a clogged filter: it can't filter out toxins properly, which can lead to a harmful build-up in your body. A clean, functioning liver plays a vital role in many bodily processes, including digestion, metabolism, immunity and hormonal balance. Regular liver cleansing can improve digestion, increase energy and even help regulate your mood.

Liver cleansing is not just a detoxification process; it's also an opportunity to reset your body. It can help reduce inflammation, improve mental clarity and strengthen your immune system. Performing a liver cleanse is taking a proactive step for your long-term health. It can help prevent liver-related diseases, such as non-alcoholic fatty liver, and contribute to increased longevity.

Finally, a liver cleanse can be an excellent starting point for a healthier lifestyle change. It can encourage you to adopt healthier eating habits, reduce your alcohol intake and adopt a regular exercise routine.

In short, liver cleansing is not just an act of caring for this vital organ, but a step towards improved overall health and a better quality of life. Herbs and/or coffee enemas can be used. See the section on preparing for dry fasting.

3.2 The Importance of a Healthy Gut for Immunity

Intestinal cleansing is not just a simple detoxification process. It is vitally important for maintaining a strong immune system. The intestine is often called the "second brain". It is a major player in our immune health. In fact, around 70% of our immune system resides in the intestine. It is therefore essential to maintain a tight, healthy intestine for optimum protection against pathogens and disease.

A healthy intestine is synonymous with a complete intestinal barrier. This barrier prevents harmful substances, such as toxins and pathogenic bacteria, from entering the bloodstream. A damaged or 'permeable' intestinal wall can lead to a range of health problems, including autoimmune disorders, by allowing unwanted substances to pass through.

The intestinal flora, or microbiota, also plays a vital role in maintaining this barrier and in the functioning of the immune system. An imbalance in the microbiota, known as dysbiosis, can lead to excessive bacterial proliferation and disrupt intestinal health. Regular, controlled intestinal cleansing can help to rebalance the intestinal flora, promoting a healthy gut and a better immune response.

It's important to remember that maintaining intestinal health isn't just about cleaning the bowels. A balanced diet rich in fibre, probiotics and prebiotics, adequate hydration, physical exercise and stress management all play a crucial role in promoting intestinal health and, by extension, immunity.

In short, a healthy gut is a pillar of immune health. A leaky gut, a balanced microbiota and attention to overall gut health are essential for preventing disease and promoting a state of general well-being.

3.3 The importance of intestinal cleansing before dry fasting

Before starting a dry fasting cure, it is crucial to prepare the body, in particular by cleansing the intestines. This step helps to eliminate toxins and optimise the benefits of fasting. Failure to cleanse the intestines before a cure can complicate it, reduce the therapeutic effects and cause pain when you come off dry fasting.

Several natural products can be used for this intestinal cleansing, each with its own beneficial properties. A naturopath specialising in dry fasting will be able to recommend these products in synergy or in combination, and a consultation to refine which preparation to adopt on a personalised basis. Here are a few suggestions for the reader, but they are not exhaustive and do not replace a consultation with a naturopath.

1. **Clay:** Clay is known for its ability to absorb toxins and help eliminate them from the body. It acts as a gentle cleanser for the intestines.
2. **Zeolite**: Zeolite is a natural mineral that can capture and eliminate heavy metals and other toxins from the body. It is often used to purify the digestive system.
3. **Silicea Med**: This silica-based food supplement helps to strengthen the intestinal walls and improve digestive health in general.
4. **Regulat:** This is a fermented concentrate of fruit, nuts and vegetables. It helps to balance intestinal flora and improve digestion.
5. **Pianto**: Pianto is a food supplement rich in nutrients and minerals, helping to revitalise and strengthen the body during the cleansing process.
6. **Neem:** Neem is a plant with detoxifying and purifying properties, often used to cleanse the digestive system.
7. **Combination of liquorice and turmeric:** Liquorice and turmeric are two herbs known for their anti-inflammatory properties and beneficial effects on intestinal health.

8. **Siberian fir resin**: This natural resin has regenerative properties and is used to strengthen and purify the intestines and is an excellent preparation for dry fasting.

Each of these products works in its own way to cleanse and regenerate the intestine, preparing it for dry fasting. It is important to choose the product or combination of products that best suits your needs and to consult a healthcare professional if you have any doubts or specific medical conditions. A clean and healthy gut before fasting not only helps to avoid discomfort, but also optimises the overall health benefits of dry fasting.

3.4 The coffee enema and its effects on health and the liver

It's a powerful detoxification process, simple and inexpensive. Coffee enemas help to cleanse the intestines, open the bile ducts, eliminate toxins from the liver, stimulate the GTS enzyme system (antioxidant enzyme), evacuate fixed acids, in particular ammoniacal nitrogen (which disrupts cellular communication and causes mental confusion), and so on.

Dr Max Gerson, a German doctor who died in 1959, promoted this method for detoxifying the body. For thousands of years, traditional medicine had advised regular cleansing of the liver. He points out that 98% of people suffering from cancers of the internal organs and other serious metabolic diseases do not die from the disease itself, but rather from the enormous overload of the liver, which is no longer able to eliminate the toxins and decomposing elements of the tumours.

- **What are the benefits of a coffee enema?**

Caffeine taken rectally increases the flow of toxin-laden bile. This helps combat flu-like symptoms and headaches. It has a beneficial effect on the lungs and skin. The elimination of free radicals is increased by 650 to 700%. No other product or medicine can compete with coffee in this respect. The enzymatic systems in the liver and small intestine are responsible for neutralising most toxins. The role of these systems is greatly enhanced by coffee enemas. They relieve nervous tension, depression and allergic symptoms, and improve circulation, immunity, cell repair and regeneration. This practice increases vitality, reduces the need to take medication and sedates severe pain. This method was used during the First World War to soothe the intense pain of the severely wounded.

An organically adapted diet and coffee enemas help to keep the intestines free of the waste products and toxins that are at the root of many illnesses, keep the liver clean and allow you to enjoy a vigorous body. The liquid from the enema that bathes the large intestine also helps to dislodge any dry matter that might stick to it. We are therefore performing two operations in one: a bile flush that will evacuate toxins and a colon cleansing. This enema, which should be kept in for between ten and 20 minutes, will prevent the toxic bile eliminated in the intestines from being reabsorbed by the intestinal capillaries into the liver (bile can normally be reabsorbed up to ten times before being eliminated in the faeces). To be filtered by the liver, the blood coming from the intestinal capillaries passes every three minutes from the intestines to the liver, carrying all the toxins collected in the body. Under the effect of caffeine, these toxins are absorbed (coffee enemas act like dialysis) and passed in the faeces. So, if we leave the enema on for 15 minutes and do it four or five times in a row, clean blood will pass to the liver, which will then get rid of the accumulated toxins. The intestines, which are also cleansed, will find it easier to eliminate the toxins once again released in the bile, etc.

The caffeine in coffee is not absorbed by the body, as it goes no further than the sigmoid colon. However, if you are allergic to caffeine, coffee enemas are not for you. Enemas should preferably be performed on an empty stomach, but in any case as far as possible from the last meal: in the morning when you wake up before breakfast, or before lunch and dinner. For people who are not used to drinking coffee, it is not advisable to do this enema in the evening, as it can disrupt sleep. But this is not always true.

- **How do I use coffee enemas?**

The essential accessory is the bock or enema bag. There are models available from chemists or various websites for a modest sum. It is advisable to use green coffee rather than black coffee, as the roasting process produces compounds that are a little uncomfortable for the body. But you can still use ground Arabica and organic black coffee. Above all, don't use instant freeze-dried coffee.

The other advantage of using green coffee is that the spasms during the session will be much weaker than with conventional coffee, as if the body had less need to get rid of them. This makes it easier to concentrate on the belly massage, and to keep going for the full 20 minutes.

- **Preparing green coffee beans**

Green coffee beans are hard, so soak them for 12 to 24 hours before use. Then dry and grind. If you don't have a coffee grinder, use a blender for one to two minutes to thoroughly pulverise the coffee beans. Use three tablespoons of green coffee or ground Arabica coffee. Bring a litre of water to the boil, add the three tablespoons of coffee and leave to infuse for 15 minutes. Then filter the mixture using an organic paper filter or a previously rinsed cotton cloth to remove any detergent and fabric softener residues. Then add fresh or lukewarm water to make 1.8 to two litres of liquid.

Allow the temperature to fall to between 37 and 40°. Then perform the enema as follows. After oiling the cannula and draining the water from the tube, gently insert the cannula into the anus. The enema bag is hung 1.5 metres from the floor. The procedure is usually started lying on the floor, on a large towel or on a protected bed. The knees are bent, the pelvis may be raised a little, and then you move to the right side (liver side), so that the liquid can spread more easily into the large intestine.

Then alternate between the right and left sides, so as to stir the interior thoroughly. When you're on your back, you can gently massage the area where the colon passes (the ascending colon is on the right side of your stomach, the transverse colon runs horizontally under your stomach, and the descending colon runs vertically down the left side of your stomach towards the exit).

Once the liquid has completely drained, the tap has been closed and the cannula removed, the aim is to hold on for between ten and 20 minutes. Some people recommend keeping the cannula in place to avoid accidental leaks. Finally, finish the session for a few minutes on your left side, so that the liquid accumulates in the descending colon, near the outlet. Note that depending on the coffee used, the urge to interrupt the session to run to the toilet will be stronger or weaker. You may also experience a few spasms of strong intensity, bordering on pain, but which generally don't last too long. Everyone has their own method for overcoming them. You can bend or pinch the tube to momentarily stop the flow of fluid, do the "puppy dog" breathing or take a slow, deep breath. In all cases, try to keep the liquid for between ten and 20 minutes.

The evacuation can then last from 15 to 30 minutes, with breaks. You can massage your stomach, rock back and forth, or put your feet up on a low stool for people who find it a little difficult to evacuate. The first thing you'll feel after washing is lightness, a gentle warmth in the belly, a slight euphoria and a sense of well-being. The famous German hydrotherapist Louis Kuhne once said: *"Only purity cures"*.

4. Personalised naturopathic consultation before dry fasting

Before starting a dry fasting cure, a consultation is essential, particularly when it includes the use of the Metatron NLS device. Here's an overview of why a consultation is necessary.

1. **Accurate assessment of your state of health.** Before starting a dry fasting cure, it is crucial to know your current state of health. The Metatron NLS device is an advanced diagnostic tool that analyses various body parameters to provide a complete picture of the patient's state of health. It can identify imbalances, deficiencies or pre-existing conditions that could affect or be affected by fasting.
2. **Personalised planning.** A naturopathic consultation can create a personalised dry fasting plan tailored to the individual's specific needs. This includes recommendations on the duration of the fast, methods of preparing for and exiting the fast, as well as advice on any dietary supplements or diet changes that may be required.
3. **Preparation and safety.** A naturopath can help prepare the body for dry fasting in a way that minimises the risks and maximises the benefits. This can include bowel cleansing strategies, a diet tailored to the individual before the fast, and advice on maintaining electrolyte balance.
4. **Post-fasting follow-up.** After the fast is over, follow-up with a naturopath is important to ensure that the transition back to a normal diet is smooth and to assess the effects of dry fasting on the body. The naturopath can adjust the therapeutic plan according to the results obtained and recovery needs.
5. **Holistic approach**: Naturopathy considers the individual as a whole, taking into account not only physical aspects but also emotional, mental and environmental factors. This holistic approach is particularly beneficial in the context of dry fasting, where body and mind are intimately linked.

In summary, a personalised naturopathic consultation, complemented by the Metatron NLS analysis, offers a thorough and safe preparation for dry fasting. It ensures that fasting is tailored to the specific needs of the individual and that it is undertaken responsibly and effectively.

5. Can I dry fast at home?

Dry fasting can be practised at home, but this requires special attention and a thorough understanding of dry fasting methods, as well as a suitable environment. Dry fasting to treat temporary ailments such as the flu, gastro-enteritis or acute pain can be beneficial if you have a good grasp of the principles of dry fasting. However, the immediate environment plays a crucial role. A natural setting, free from pollution and away from food temptations, is ideal for undertaking a long dry fast and has nothing to do with short dry fasts.

It is essential to recognise the importance of the internal changes brought about by dry fasting. This process is not just a break from food, but an opportunity for profound physical and spiritual transformation. Changing location during the fast can facilitate this metamorphosis by establishing new positive intentions and encouraging a review of lifestyle and diet.

Taking part in a dry fast in a dedicated centre has significant advantages. The atmosphere is often happier, more reassuring and conducive to mutual support, thereby increasing the benefits of fasting. As well as offering emotional security, group support helps to save energy, leaving more resources available for regeneration, detoxification and bodily renewal. What's more, fasting in a group allows you to better manage any emotions or pain that may arise, benefiting from the collective experience and sound advice.

For those who have never experienced dry fasting, embarking on this adventure alone can be complex and sometimes disconcerting when faced with the emergence of unfamiliar sensations. Adequate preparation over a period of a month or more is advisable if you are to approach fasting calmly and safely, particularly if you have any specific medical conditions. In such cases, prolonged fasting of seven to ten days may be recommended under supervision and with appropriate support.

It is therefore crucial to weigh up the advantages and disadvantages of practising dry fasting alone at home. Although it may be suitable for short, one-off fasts, the experience and effectiveness of dry fasting can be greatly enhanced in a group context and under professional supervision. According to observations and testimonies, the effectiveness of group dry fasting can exceed that of fasting alone by 40-70%. The decision to fast at home or in a group should therefore be carefully considered, taking into account your own abilities, health and personal well-being goals.

6. The value of genetic testing to determine your ideal diet according to your APOE profile before and after therapeutic dry fasting by Michel Deladoey, naturopath

Introduction

In the field of nutrition and preventive health, genetic tests such as those which determine the APOE profile from saliva or blood samples are becoming increasingly important in therapeutic fasting cures, and your fasting companions need to cover these subjects in their preventive pre-fasting and especially post-fasting aliemntation. Apolipoprotein E (APOE) plays a crucial role in lipid metabolism and is strongly associated with the prevention of several chronic diseases. Understanding one's APOE profile can therefore help personalise diets to improve overall health and prevent specific diseases.

What is APOE?

APOE is a protein involved in lipoprotein metabolism, essential for the transport and metabolism of cholesterol and triglycerides.

Three main alleles of this protein – E2, E3, and E4 – and their genetic combinations (or genotypes) can significantly affect health.

APOE alleles and genotypes

- **E2 (ε2)**: Associated with lower levels of LDL cholesterol and a reduced risk of heart disease, but may increase the risk of neurological disease in some cases.
- **E3 (ε3)**: The most common allele, considered neutral in the context of lipid metabolism-related diseases.
- **E4 (ε4)**: Increases the risk of cardiovascular disease, Alzheimer's disease, and may negatively influence cholesterol metabolism.

Objectives of APOE profiling

APOE genetic profiling aims to:

- **Prevent heart disease**: by adapting lipid intake according to genotype.
- **Controlling the risk of diabetes**: with personalised diets that take glucose metabolism into account.
- **Manage high blood pressure**: by adjusting salt and saturated fat intake.
- **Reduce the risk of Alzheimer's disease**: especially for carriers of the E4 allele, by means of diets enriched with antioxidants and low in saturated fats.
- **Controlling excess weight**: by optimising the diet to improve basal metabolic rate according to APOE genotype.
- **Prevent lung disease**: by avoiding aggravating substances identified by the genetic profile.

Benefits of genetic testing before dry fasting

1. **Identifying potential risks**: Some APOE genotypes may be more susceptible to imbalances during dry fasting, increasing the risk of complications.
2. **Optimising the benefits of dry fasting**: By knowing your APOE profile, you can adapt the duration and nature of fasting to maximise the positive effects on your health.
3. **Preparing the body**: Adjust your diet before dry fasting to prepare the metabolism, in particular by adjusting macronutrient intakes.

The benefits of genetic testing after therapeutic dry fasting

After a dry fast, the body is in a state of readaptation. Genetic testing then offers significant advantages:

1. **Personalising the refeeding**: Based on the APOE profile, the refeeding phase can be adjusted to avoid dietary imbalances. An apo E2, for example, would be advised to follow a very low-carbohydrate diet, or even a ketogenic diet, rich in animal protein, whereas an E4 could be improved by eating more plants and fewer meat products.
2. **Evaluating the benefits of fasting**: The test can help to understand how fasting has affected lipid and general metabolism, depending on the genetic profile.
3. **Adapting the diet over the long term**: Genetic information can be used to design a sustainable diet that prevents disease based on the results of fasting and the APOE profile.

Genetic testing to determine the APOE profile is a proactive approach to preventive medicine and personalised nutrition. Before and after a dry fast, knowing your APOE profile means you can adapt your diet precisely to improve your overall health and reduce the risk of chronic disease. This genetic-based personalisation is at the frontier of modern nutrition and predictive medicine, offering an optimal strategy for maintaining long-term optimal health.

Targeted dietary recommendations

Apolipoprotein E (ApoE) is essential for lipid metabolism and influences various aspects of health, including coagulation, immunity and heavy metal detoxification. APOE polymorphisms, in particular the E2, E3 and E4 alleles, have a significant impact on the risk of developing certain diseases and on the way the body reacts to different diets.

ApoE genotypes and their implications

E2 (ε2)

- **Genotype:** E2/E2, E2/E3
- **Risks:**
  - Reduces LDL cholesterol levels, thereby lowering the risk of cardiovascular disease.
  - May increase the risk of type III hyperlipoproteinemia (accumulation of cholesterol).

- **Food recommendations:**
  - **Fats:** 20-25% of total intake, with a preference for monounsaturated and polyunsaturated fats (olive oil, avocados). Limit saturated fats and avoid trans fats.
  - **Protein:** 25% of intake, favouring lean and vegetable sources (legumes, fish).
  - **Carbohydrates:** low and very low glycaemic index (vegetables, very few wholegrain cereals or slow carbohydrates max 10%).

  - **Physical activity:** Balance between aerobic and anaerobic activity, with a focus on gentle activities that do not increase lipid pressure too much.

E3 (ε3)

- **Genotype:** E3/E3 (most common)
- **Risks:**
  - No marked specific risks or benefits; risk of disease related to the general population.

- **Food recommendations:**
  - **Fats:** 25% of intake, focusing on monounsaturated and polyunsaturated fats. Avoid trans fats.
  - **Protein:** 20% to 40% of intake, with a preference for combined proteins, i.e. animal and vegetable proteins, fish and eggs.
  - **Carbohydrates:** medium to low quantities, choosing low-glycaemic index carbohydrates rich in fibre (fruit, vegetables, wholegrain cereals).
  - **Physical activity:** A balance of 50% aerobic (walking, cycling) and 50% anaerobic (weight training, sprints).

E4 (ε4)

- **Genotype:** E4/E4, E3/E4
- **Risks:**
  - Increases the risk of Alzheimer's disease and cardiovascular disease.
  - May alter cholesterol metabolism, increasing LDL and lowering HDL. Monitor liver health and encourage regular or intermittent fasting.

- **Food recommendations:**
  - **Fats:** Reduce fat intake to 10-20%, minimising saturated fats and eliminating trans fats. Increase sources of omega-3 (oily fish, flaxseed).
  - **Protein:** 25%, favouring lean sources and fish rich in omega-3.
  - **Carbohydrates:** medium to low, with an emphasis on fibre and slow, complex carbohydrates (vegetables, legumes, wholegrain cereals).
  - **Physical activity:** More aerobic (60%) to improve lipid profile, with 40% anaerobic to maintain muscle mass.

General Recommendations for Other Genotypes

E2/E4

- **Risks:** Combines certain risks of E2 and E4, particularly in terms of lipid levels.

- **Food recommendations:**
  - **Fats:** 25%, concentrating on monounsaturated fats and increasing omega-3s.
  - **Protein:** 20-25%, from a variety of sources including vegetables and fish.
  - **Carbohydrates:** low to moderate, giving priority to complex carbohydrates and fibre.
  - **Physical activity:** Balance between aerobic activity for the heart and weak anaerobic activity to maintain muscle mass.
  - **Phytotherapeutic support**. Ginkgo, biloba.

Frequency of alleles in the world population according to available scientific studies

- **ε2**: 5-10%
- **ε3**: 65-80%
- **ε4**: 10-20%

Frequency of genotypes

Genotypes are formed by the combination of these alleles. The frequency of genotypes in the general population is approximately:

1. **ε2/ε2**: 1% or less
2. **ε2/ε3**: 10-15
3. **ε2/ε4**: 2-5
4. **ε3/ε3**: 50-70
5. **ε3/ε4**: 20-30% of the value
6. **ε4/ε4**: 1-5

Precise details by genotype

- **ε2/ε2**: This genotype is quite rare, representing less than 1% of the population. It is often associated with lower cholesterol levels and a reduced risk of coronary heart disease, but a higher risk of lipoprotein-related diseases, such as type III hyperlipoproteinaemia.
- **ε2/ε3**: Present in around 10-15% of the population, this genotype is associated with generally favourable lipid profiles and a moderately reduced risk of cardiovascular disease and Alzheimer's compared with ε3/ε3.
- **ε2/ε4**: This genotype is less common, accounting for 2-5% of the population. The effects of ε2 and ε4 can offset

each other, leading to variable lipid profiles and a more moderate risk of cardiovascular disease and Alzheimer's.

- **ε3/ε3**: The most common, this genotype represents around 50-70% of the population and is often used as a reference in genetic risk studies. It is associated with a standard risk of cardiovascular disease and Alzheimer's.
- **ε3/ε4**: Present in around 20-30% of the population, this genotype is associated with an increased risk of Alzheimer's disease and cardiovascular disorders, compared with ε3/ε3.
- **ε4/ε4**: This genotype is rare (1-5% of the population) and is most strongly associated with a high risk of Alzheimer's disease and cardiovascular disease.

Important notes

- These frequencies can vary significantly according to ethnic origin and geographical region. For example, the ε4 allele is less common in East Asia, but more common in the indigenous peoples of America and sub-Saharan Africa.
- The risk factors associated with each genotype are influenced by many other factors, including lifestyle, diet, physical activity and other genes.

Which phytotherapeutic remedies and foods to choose according to genotype

Specific for Apo E ε2
Food and Mineral supplements for Apo E ε2

1. **Omega-3 Fatty Acids (EPA and DHA)**
   - **Benefits:** Helps regulate the lipid profile by reducing triglycerides and increasing

HDL ('good' cholesterol). They also have anti-inflammatory effects that may benefit cardiovascular health.
- **Sources:** Fish oil, krill oil, or seaweed for a vegetarian option.
- **Use:** Supplements of 1-2 grams a day or as recommended by a health professional.

2. **Soluble fibres**
   - **Benefits:** Helps reduce the absorption of dietary cholesterol in the intestine and regulate blood lipid levels.
   - **Sources:** Psyllium, oats, apples, barley.
   - **Use:** Incorporate into the diet or take as a supplement, around 5-10 grams a day.

3. **Niacin (Vitamin B3)**
   - **Benefits:** Can help increase HDL and reduce triglycerides and LDL ('bad') cholesterol.
   - **Use:** Supplements under medical supervision to avoid side effects at high doses.

4. **Magnesium**
   - **Benefits:** Important for more than 300 biochemical reactions in the body, including lipid metabolism. It can help regulate blood pressure and heart rate.
   - **Sources:** Green leafy vegetables, nuts, whole grains and food supplements.
   - **Use:** 200-400mg per day as recommended by a healthcare professional.

5. **Vitamin E**
   - **Benefits:** A powerful antioxidant that may help protect low-density lipoproteins (LDL) from oxidation, a risk factor for cardiovascular disease.

- **Sources:** Vegetable oils, nuts, seeds and food supplements.
- **Usage:** 15mg (22 IU) per day or as recommended by a healthcare professional.

6. **Coenzyme Q10 (CoQ10)**
   - **Benefits:** Important antioxidant that helps protect cells against oxidative stress; supports mitochondrial function and may improve cellular energy.
   - **Use:** Recommended food supplements, particularly for those taking statins or who need mitochondrial support.

7. **Turmeric (Curcumin)**
   - **Benefits:** Anti-inflammatory and antioxidant, may help reduce the risk of cardiovascular and neurodegenerative diseases.
   - **Use:** Used in cooking, as a food supplement or as a tea.

8. **Vitamin D**
   - **Benefits:** Contributes to bone health and immune function; studies also suggest a role in reducing inflammation and protecting against certain chronic diseases.
   - **Sources:** Sun exposure, fortified foods and food supplements.
   - **Usage:** 800-2000 IU per day or as recommended by a healthcare professional.

9. **Antioxidants (Polyphenols, Vitamin C)**
   - **Benefits:** Helps protect against oxidative stress and inflammation, supporting cardiovascular health.

- **Sources:** Fruit, vegetables, green tea, dark chocolate and food supplements.
- **Use:** Include a variety of sources in the diet and consider supplements if necessary.

Food and Mineral supplements for Apo E ε3

1. **Omega-3 Fatty Acids (EPA and DHA)**
   - **Benefits:** Contributes to cardiovascular health by reducing inflammation and triglycerides and improving the lipid profile.
   - **Sources:** Fish oil, krill oil, or seaweed for a vegetarian option.
   - **Use:** Supplements of 1-2 grams a day or as recommended by a health professional.

2. **Vitamin D**
   - **Benefits:** Essential for bone health and immune function, and plays a role in reducing inflammation and protecting against certain chronic diseases.
   - **Sources:** Sun exposure, fortified foods and food supplements.
   - **Usage:** 800-2000 IU per day or as recommended by a healthcare professional.

3. **Magnesium**
   - **Benefits:** Important for more than 300 biochemical reactions in the body, helps regulate blood pressure and heart rate, and supports energy metabolism.
   - **Sources:** Green leafy vegetables, nuts, whole grains and food supplements.
   - **Use:** 200-400mg per day as recommended by a healthcare professional.

4. **Soluble fibres**
    - **Benefits:** Helps regulate blood glucose and cholesterol levels, improving digestive and cardiovascular health.
    - **Sources:** Psyllium, oats, apples, barley.
    - **Use:** Incorporate into the diet or take as a supplement, around 5-10 grams a day.

5. **Vitamin C**
    - **Benefits:** Antioxidant that helps protect cells against free radical damage, supports the immune system and collagen production.
    - **Sources:** citrus fruits, berries, kiwis, peppers and food supplements.
    - **Use:** 500-1000mg per day or as recommended by a healthcare professional

6. **Coenzyme Q10 (CoQ10)**
    - **Benefits:** Important antioxidant that helps protect cells against oxidative stress; supports mitochondrial function and may improve cellular energy.
    - **Use:** Recommended food supplements, particularly for those taking statins or who need mitochondrial support.

7. **Polyphenols (particularly those found in green tea and turmeric)**
    - **Benefits:** Powerful antioxidants, may help reduce the risk of chronic disease by reducing inflammation and protecting against oxidative stress.
    - **Sources:** Green tea (catechins), turmeric (curcumin), berries, dark chocolate.
    - **Use:** Include in the diet or take as a supplement as recommended.

8. **Probiotics**
   - **Benefits:** Support digestive health, may help maintain a healthy balance of intestinal flora, which is beneficial for immunity and overall metabolism.
   - **Sources:** yoghurt, kefir, fermented products and food supplements.
   - **Use:** Follow the dosage recommendations on supplement products.

9. **Vitamin E**
   - **Benefits:** A powerful antioxidant that may help protect low-density lipoproteins (LDL) from oxidation, a risk factor for cardiovascular disease.
   - **Sources:** Vegetable oils, nuts, seeds and food supplements.
   - **Usage:** 15mg (22 IU) per day or as recommended by a healthcare professional.

10. **Selenium**
    - **Benefits:** An essential mineral that plays a key role in metabolism and antioxidant functions, supporting immune function and thyroid health.
    - **Sources:** Brazil nuts, seafood, whole grains and food supplements.
    - **Usage:** 55-200 micrograms per day as recommended by a healthcare professional.

11. **Lawyer**
    - **Active ingredients:** Monounsaturated fatty acids, polyphenols
    - **Benefits:** Improves lipid profile, antioxidant.
    - **Use:** Regularly included in the diet to support heart and brain health.

12. **Blueberries**
    - **Active ingredients:** Anthocyanins, flavonoids

  - **Benefits:** Antioxidant, may help improve cognitive function and protect against oxidative stress.
  - **Use:** Add regularly to the diet.

13. **Almonds**
  - **Active ingredients:** Vitamin E, monounsaturated fatty acids
  - **Benefits:** Antioxidant, improves lipid profile, supports brain health.
  - **Use:** Consume a small portion regularly to benefit from its protective effects.

Specific for Apo E ε4

People with the ε4 genotype have an increased risk of cardiovascular disease and Alzheimer's. In addition to the above plants, the following may be particularly beneficial:

1. **Ginkgo biloba**
  - **Benefits:** Improves cerebral circulation, has neuroprotective effects, may help improve memory and cognitive function.
  - **Use:** Food supplements as recommended by a health professional.

2. **Berries (blueberries, raspberries, blackberries)**
  - **Active ingredients:** Anthocyanins
  - **Benefits:** Powerful antioxidants, may help improve memory and cognitive function, reduce inflammation.
  - **Use:** Regularly included in the diet.

3. **Walnut (Juglans regia)**
  - **Active ingredients:** Omega-3 fatty acids, polyphenols

   - **Benefits:** Supports brain health, improves lipid profile.
   - **Use:** Include a handful of nuts in your daily diet.

4. **Fir resin (Abies spp.)**
   - **Active ingredients:** Resin acids, terpenoids
   - **Benefits:** Powerful antioxidant, may help protect cells against oxidative stress; has potential beneficial effects on cardiovascular health thanks to its anti-inflammatory properties, positive effect on oxidised LDL high natural level
   - **Use:** Can be used in the form of liquid food extracts.

5. **Coenzyme Q10 (CoQ10)**
   - **Benefits:** Important antioxidant that helps protect cells against oxidative stress; supports mitochondrial function and may improve cellular energy; particularly beneficial for the heart and brain.
   - **Use:** Recommended dietary supplements, particularly for those taking statins or who need increased mitochondrial support.

Conclusion on these genetic tests

Determining the ApoE genotype through genetic testing offers a unique opportunity to personalise the diet and avoid dietary errors to optimise health according to individual predispositions. Each ApoE genotype has its own specificities, which can be adjusted by dietary modifications and a suitable exercise plan to minimise the risk of disease and improve general well-being. The test should be carried out by your doctor or naturopath, provided they are familiar with this branch of dietary and morphobenetic medicine.

CHAPTER 12

Method of practising ten-day dry fasting

Happiness is about living in the moment, enjoying every minute and accepting with gratitude all that life has to offer. Even in adversity, it gives us the strength to overcome anything. Print this sentence during your dry fast.

1. How it works: what happens during the fast?

- **Day 1**

To tackle the first day of dry fasting, psychological preparation is essential. It's important to repeat positive statements to yourself, such as: "Everything will be fine, I feel fit, I'm looking forward to the coming days, I can stop fasting without risk at any time if necessary". If you are well prepared, surrounded and in a calm environment, this first day will go smoothly. During this first day, it is normal to feel thirsty and slightly weak, as the sugar level in the body drops slightly. To save energy, it is advisable to go to bed early, limit talking and practise relaxing activities such as abdominal massage, breathing exercises, yoga and meditation. Weight loss on this day generally varies between 0.5 and 2 kg.

Dry fasting, even for a single day, has been recognised for its health benefits, as confirmed by a Nobel Prize. From the very first day, the therapeutic mechanisms of autophagy are activated, leading to the cleansing and recycling of dysfunctional elements in the cells. This process protects the body from ageing, preserves DNA integrity and can even contribute to rejuvenation by encouraging the creation of new cells. In fasting mode, the cell activates its defence mechanism and switches to energy-saving mode. These processes demonstrate the effectiveness of dry fasting not only for weight loss, but also for strengthening cellular functions and promoting longevity. The key to successful fasting lies in mental and physical preparation, as well as respect for your body and its limits.

- **Day 2**

The aim is to keep my mind occupied in an intelligent way and to embark on a personal inner journey, by putting myself in regeneration and inner healing mode. I put myself in my inner bubble and see myself as a hero or as someone on a path of initiation. I monitor my energy expenditure and leave myself time to do nothing. I make my own little programme for the day. Sometimes you may feel dizzy, have a headache or feel uncomfortable in your stomach. From day 2, all glycogen stocks are depleted in the liver and muscles, so you have to be vigilant for fatigue. The body then goes into ketosis. Don't be afraid of these symptoms of tiredness: it's the body's endogenous restructuring and cleansing process that is triggered. You need to walk, move around and get some fresh air. Also take the biotherapies suggested. In the evening, before going to bed, do some relaxation exercises or meditation, whatever the centre suggests.

It is from this day that cell biosynthesis begins, which is similar to the biosynthesis of plant cells. The human cell is completely free to absorb carbon dioxide and nitrogen from the air! In this case, the problem of essential amino acids disappears.

Cell biosynthesis is qualitatively improved, producing such substances by itself and in quantities that it cannot produce on a diet! This determines the complete internal nutrition of a fasting person. It is known that carbon from carbon dioxide, converted into carbon from organic substances, gives two molecules of oxygen, plus the extra energy that is formed when carbon is restored. This is what happens during ketoacidosis. If you fast cyclically, then you are continually activating endogenous biosynthesis, whereas with simple food, the body can survive much better than with saturation with balanced proteins and other elements.

If we briefly summarise the beneficial effects of the abovementioned physiological mechanisms on the body, this will result in the repair of the hereditary apparatus, and even of DNA, with improved methylation. In addition, there will be a restoration of the body's enzyme systems (immunity and digestion will be improved), a restoration of cell membranes (they take on the form of fasting cells and the restoration of cell barriers occurs), an increase in the number and quality of cells in the gastrointestinal tract, as well as the destruction of excess fat and cells. https://www.ncbi.nlm.nih.gov/pmc/articles/PMC9065201/

From the second day onwards, the anti-inflammatory and immunostimulant mechanisms of dry fasting are activated. As a result, illnesses such as acute respiratory infections and influenza or Covid can be completely cured. Three days for flu seems to be the best choice. Purification of the intestines and blood vessels begins on the second day.

https://news.mit.edu/2018/fasting-boosts-stem-cells-regenerative-capacity-0503

Make sure you massage your abdomen and spine if you can.

- **Day 3**

That day, for example, is the minimum required to treat a flu infection, i.e. three full nights. Most people who undergo dry fasting will generally develop acidosis. A very important moment in dry fasting is the acidotic crisis which occurs after the switch to endogenous nutrition and which may give rise to some symptoms. Don't be afraid of feeling unwell during this period, as everything will be fine afterwards.

For beginners in dry fasting, this generally occurs over three days. An acidotic crisis occurs when the concentration of ketone bodies (products of the incomplete decomposition of triglycerides or fats) increases and the transformation process is saturated.

During this period, you will feel unwell: typical signs of intoxication are felt. However, as soon as ketone bodies start to be used, their concentration stops increasing and, as ketone bodies are high-energy compounds, the synthesis of new amino acids begins on them, as on fuel, which can lead to tissue regeneration.

The regeneration process can occur with intense pain, and you should be prepared and expect this. In the early stages of dry fasting, the acidotic crisis may occur on the third or even second day after the start of dry fasting. Body type can also play a role. A sanguine person and a neuroarthritic person will not have the same signs at the same time. A slimmer person may need fewer days to reach these elimination crises. This varies.

With each new dry fast, the crisis occurs sooner. The quicker the crisis passes, the more time is left to renew the body. At this point, there may be an acetone smell in the mouth, nausea, dizziness, shortness of breath and a feeling of weakness. Hunger is reduced and thirst is tolerable.

Blood pressure varies according to the characteristics of each individual's body. There is no need to be afraid of these phenomena, as the body adapts to the new conditions of vital activity and the symptoms are somewhat exacerbated. The best thing to do during this period is to take calm, slow walks in nature. Self-massage of the abdomen, breathing, yoga and massage are a plus.

Fasting is the process of increasing physiological regeneration, the renewal of all cells and their molecular and chemical composition. An interesting fact is that the biochemical changes during fasting and reparative regeneration are very similar.

In both cases, there are two phases: destruction (catabolism) and restoration (anabolism). In both cases, destruction is characterised by the predominance of the degradation of proteins and nucleic acids over their synthesis, by the shift of pH to the acidic side, by acidosis and other phenomena. The recovery phase is also characterised in both cases by the predominance of the synthesis of nucleic acids over their decomposition, and the return of the pH to a neutral state.

According to regeneration theory, it is known that an increase in the destruction phase leads to an increase in the recovery phase. It is therefore reasonable to consider therapeutic dry fasting as a natural factor in stimulating physiological regeneration.

Therapeutic dry fasting is based on a general biological process leading to the renewal and rejuvenation of tissues throughout the body. In modern humans, under unfavourable ecological conditions, the physiological mechanisms of regeneration function incompletely. During therapeutic dry fasting, the body is cleansed and the regeneration mechanisms begin to function naturally. As soon as the process of voluntary intoxication ends, the body rejects anything foreign.

Everything that can be regenerated is like a spring that springs back to life as soon as the oppression is removed. Everything that is regenerated loves purity, cyclicality and dosage. Post-fasting excess for regenerated systems is as destructive as uncleanliness and what is not fresh. During dry fasting, the first thing that happens is that diseased, pathological tissues are destroyed, triggering a universal mechanism in the body for healing wounds using the internal cell reserve, the stromal cells of the bone marrow. This is one of the main mechanisms for eliminating the consequences of any injury.

After cessation of dry fasting, there is an increase in regeneration processes in the bloodstream of the bone marrow (an increase in mitotically dividing cells etc.). Indicators of regeneration of the haematopoietic system in the peripheral blood (e.g. reticulocytes) are generally three times higher than the initial figures. But most importantly, bone marrow stromal cells appear in greater numbers than usual. These cells can be transformed into any type of other cell by being found in the appropriate area of the body. The stromal cells begin to flow into the damaged area when they receive the appropriate signal from the central nervous system. Once in the damaged area, they are transformed into the cells that are missing from the damaged tissue, under the action of certain signalling molecules. It has been established that dry fasting restores and even increases brain pyramidal cells and boosts the famous BDNF. From the third day onwards, the renewal of tissue fluid begins and the partial restoration of the gastrointestinal epithelium.

- **Day 4**

During dry fasting, a fascinating process takes place within the body, characterised by a series of normal physiological reactions. One of the first observations is the variation in blood pressure, which may decrease or increase, with a rise in body temperature. This rise in temperature can sometimes manifest itself as shivering or even fever, depending on various factors such as the fasting person's physical condition, the nature of any pre-existing illnesses, as well as their sex and age.

A remarkable feature of dry fasting is the way in which every cell in the body reacts in the absence of water. They enter a state of internal combustion of toxins, temporarily metamorphosing into veritable mini-furnaces or mini-reactors. This internal reaction can be perceived by fasters as a sensation of heat or, paradoxically, of cooling, without it being necessary to measure this temperature by conventional means.

The importance of this rise in temperature cannot be underestimated, as it plays a crucial role in the body's defence mechanisms. In addition to the intensive production of antibodies, high temperature inhibits the vital activity of microbes and encourages their elimination. It also stimulates lymphocytes, boosting their ability to phagocytose microbes. In addition, a high body temperature speeds up blood circulation and increases the activity of the secretory and metabolic organs, helping to clean the body effectively.

In my own experience of dry fasting, I have observed that certain cells, including cancer cells, completely cease their vital functions at a specific temperature. After the fourth day of fasting, the epithelium of the gastrointestinal tract begins to regenerate and the liver is thoroughly cleansed.

The practice of dry fasting also opens the door to interesting experiments with cold water, which, if well tolerated, can lead to walking barefoot in snow or dew, taking cold showers or even walking naked in nature. As well as cooling the body, these activities play a part in stabilising the fasting person's condition, virtually ruling out the possibility of a cold.

This dry fasting course highlights the body's extraordinary capacity to purify and regenerate itself autonomously, revealing the unexplored potential of our own biological systems in the face of health challenges.

- **Day 5**

On the fifth day of dry fasting, a particularly powerful therapeutic phase is revealed, characterised by a marked intensification of the body's anti-inflammatory and immunostimulant mechanisms. This period is typified by a twofold benefit for the immune system: not only are old and damaged cells eliminated, but blood stem cells are also stimulated, thereby promoting cellular renewal of the immune system. Hunger forces these cells to consume their nutrient reserves, causing them also to 'eat' the old, failing immune cells. This autophagy triggers a signalling cascade that activates the blood stem cells, beginning a process of regeneration through division and the production of new, high-quality leukocytes.

During this period, it's not uncommon for chronic illnesses, even those previously unrecognised, to begin to worsen. The organs most affected may begin to ache, reminding us of the importance of preparing our bodies and minds for this intense healing process. In the face of these manifestations, it is essential to practise gratitude towards our body for its hard work.

Symptoms such as nausea may occur, and various strategies can be employed to deal with them, such as abdominal massage, applying cold to the liver area or using a hot water bottle. If you find it difficult to walk, resting in a calm, cool environment while listening to classical or vibrating music can be beneficial.

With the internal struggle against the various ailments, a rise in body temperature is often observed, accompanied by sensations of heat. Blood pressure may also fluctuate. It is advisable to adopt cold water treatments, expose yourself to fresh air as much as possible, wearing light clothing or removing clothing depending on the weather conditions, explore the biotherapies available and take it easy. If possible, going barefoot in the snow is an invigorating experience.

The fasting person may experience insomnia, increased thirst and variations in blood pressure. Each dry fasting experience is unique, reflecting the diversity of individual reactions to the process. Despite these challenges, day five marks a significant turning point in the treatment of many illnesses, whether in their acute or worsening phase. Let's innovate by considering complementary approaches to maximise the therapeutic potential of this day, such as practising meditation to calm the mind, exploring deep breathing techniques to improve cellular oxygenation, and perhaps incorporating guided visualisation sessions to support the internal healing process and strengthen the mind-body connection.

- **Day 6**

The sixth day of dry fasting is often seen as a turning point, when the mental and physical challenge reaches its peak. At this stage, increased thirst prompts the desire to moisten the mouth, although this can, paradoxically, intensify the sensation of dryness and thirst. Sleep can be drastically reduced, sometimes to just two hours a night, and a general tiredness becomes apparent for all to see, marking a growing desire to end the fasting period.

It is precisely at these difficult times that strength of will and a positive frame of mind become crucial. The practice of relaxation is an essential tool for sustaining the determination to carry on. It is essential to recognise the invaluable experience that this ordeal represents, contributing to an increase in self-respect. Every bit of progress should be celebrated, because even if the fast is not completed, the benefits in terms of mental strength and vigour of life are considerable.

The sixth day also brings with it heightened sensory acuity, particularly in the sense of smell, making certain previously neglected odours particularly pronounced. Pain may appear in the area of the sacrum and lower back, and vision may deteriorate.

It is generally between the sixth and seventh day that the active elimination of toxins and waste intensifies, manifesting itself in dark urine and general discomfort due to the release of accumulated toxins. These symptoms indicate that the internal cleansing process is underway, underlining the importance of enduring these discomforts, rejoicing in the body's ability to purify itself and understanding that all natural healing often involves a phase of aggravation.

Apoptosis, the process of programmed cell death, accelerates, playing a key role in maintaining homeostasis and preventing cellular dysfunction that could lead to internal chaos. Dry fasting helps to combat the accumulation of 'calorie-rich waste', a source of disease and premature ageing, by promoting cell renewal and purification of vital organs.

To help you get through this demanding period, it is advisable to adopt the relaxation techniques offered at your centre, such as massages, the Schuman plateau and therapeutic blankets. This will make it easier to sleep and help maintain motivation to keep going. Dry fasting, despite its challenges, is presented as a promising method for significantly improving quality of life, marking the start of a profound regeneration of the body as early as the sixth day.

- **Day 7**

The seventh day of the dry fast marks a crucial stage both physically and spiritually, because you can experience both the challenges and the profound benefits of this practice. Reaching this milestone is in itself a remarkable achievement, signifying that you are part of a select group capable of overcoming considerable obstacles. This sense of pride is well-deserved, because not only do few people reach this stage, it's also the moment when anti-inflammatory biological mechanisms kick in, ushering in a potentially most healing phase.

During this period, the body undergoes an intense purification and renewal of vital energy. It is not uncommon to experience unusual or symbolic dreams, perhaps reflecting a process of releasing negative or pathological energies, such as evil spells or the evil eye. On a physical level, this day brings tangible relief, emotional recuperation and general stabilisation, with regulation of blood pressure and intensification of the purification process, visible in the dark brown colour of the urine. To support this purification, practices such as vacuum massage, as well as self-massage of the abdomen and spine, are recommended on waking.

Dry fasting is recognised for its spiritual virtues, acting as a powerful form of purification from physical impurities and negative energies. The individual's will and intention are refined and intensified, which explains why many spiritual leaders, priests, ascetics and philosophers include fasting in their practice, for its energetic and spiritual benefits. According to various traditions, particularly in yoga, fasting helps to cleanse the energy channels and chakras, encouraging a deeper connection with nature and a positive state of mind. This purification can also play a key role in the preparation of spiritual, shamanic or magical rituals.

Interestingly, fasting can be seen as an effective means of eliminating not only physical toxins but also negative energies, making it unlikely that curses or other negative influences will persist after a seven-day fasting period. Even for those who are sceptical about immaterial aspects such as spirituality and energy, fasting offers tangible benefits by often eliminating the underlying causes of illness, where chemical drugs may fail or even make the situation worse.

To calm the body and mind during this difficult seventh day, it can be beneficial to engage in meditative or deep relaxation activities, listen to soothing music or practise breathing exercises to improve well-being and strengthen resilience in the face of the challenges of fasting. In short, the seventh day is an invitation to fully embrace the inner and outer transformations brought about by dry fasting, paving the way for healing and spiritual upliftment.

- **Day 8**

On the eighth day of dry fasting, the body and mind enter a phase of profound transformation, almost marking the end of a liberating journey. An unexpected sense of well-being and contentment begins to emerge, a sign that the internal healing mechanisms have been fully activated. During this period, sensations such as an unpleasant taste and smell in the mouth may occur, while nasal breathing becomes easier. Variations in pulse rate, increased temperature, nausea, weakness, dizziness and loose stools are all signs of the intensive cleansing process underway, particularly of the liver, digestive and lymphatic systems.

To break new ground in understanding what happens in the body on the eighth day, it is fascinating to consider the research reported in the journal *Cell Metabolism* on how fasting influences vascular health. Scientists have discovered that fasting activates the waste elimination system in macrophages, the immune cells involved in atherosclerosis, which is inflammation of the arterial walls. This self-digestion process breaks down and eliminates molecular debris, significantly reducing the risk of atherosclerosis by promoting vascular cleansing.

At this stage, pain in the mammary glands, the uterus in women, or the prostate in men, can signal therapeutic action on benign tumours and the purification of blood vessels. This illustrates the body's remarkable capacity for self-regeneration and detoxification, even in the most sensitive areas.

To support and maximise well-being during this critical phase, gentle, regenerative practices are recommended. Resting in a cool, calm place, practising self-massage, yoga, Schumann therapy, ito thermie or even taking a cold shower if tolerated, can all contribute to the feeling of comfort. Nature walks, strength permitting, offer a valuable opportunity to reconnect with the environment, breathe in fresh air and support the body's revitalisation.

Add to this the idea of incorporating deep breathing and meditation practices to encourage inner calm and emotional balance. These activities can not only help manage physical weakness and detoxification symptoms, but also strengthen spiritual connection and promote holistic healing.

In short, the eighth day of dry fasting is a special time to celebrate the resilience of the body and mind, while continuing to actively support the healing and purification process. It is essential to remain attentive to the body's signals, to adapt one's activities according to one's capacities, and to commit oneself fully to this transformative experience with patience and gratitude.

- **Day 9**

Based on my experience, I believe that this day is one of the most important in the treatment and can have a significant curative effect on the second acidosis crisis which usually occurs. If you have reached this point, try to put all your efforts, patience and willpower to the test, to get through this crisis as well as possible. On this day, all the therapeutic mechanisms reach their peak, especially during the night. It's between midnight and 5am that the body's main treatment takes place, and that's when there are the fewest toxins in circulation. Whereas during the first two stages of fasting, autolysis of body tissues was the only source of nourishment, during the second acidotic crisis, autolysis acts more like a natural surgeon.

The most important thing in all types of fasting is to pass through the second acidotic crisis, in which the activation of all the body's defences is stronger, helping to cure many incurable diseases. If we are speaking figuratively about the very great significance of these crises, then if the first acidotic crisis eliminates the stem of the disease, the second destroys the root of the disease.

By passing this day, it is possible to effectively treat infertility and certain autoimmune pathologies, for example. The large quantity of sex hormones that invade the blood during fasting leads to a sharp increase in sexual desire. Contrary to popular belief, hunger does not suppress sexuality; on the contrary, it sharpens it. The hormonal background is normalised, with complete maturation of the follicles and elimination of ovarian dysfunction.

A group of women aged between 22 and 25 during the Muslim Ramadan was examined to determine the effect of fasting on progesterone and prolactin content in blood plasma, as well as on women's reproductive physiology. The results showed that plasma prolactin levels fell in 80% of the women, while progesterone levels remained unchanged. This study proves the importance of fasting in the treatment of infertility caused by increased prolactin content. When prolactin levels fall during fasting, a woman's natural ability to have children is restored. Few women suffer from absolute sterility, infertility being the result and consequence of certain illnesses and often of an excess of toxins.

2. Think smart during dry fasting

1. Be happy and cheerful in all circumstances, thinking only of joy, happiness and gratitude.
2. Follow the recommendations given day by day and everything will be fine. Don't hesitate to contact me privately via WhatsApp during the cure if anything goes wrong or if you have any concerns. You can also contact a referee with expertise in dry fasting.
3. Dry fasting takes a lot of mental strength to keep going, but you'll be proud of what you've achieved.
4. Never try to compare yourself to others – everyone has their own pace and their own story.

5. Be aware that as the days go by, fatigue sets in and depends on your degree of intoxication. If you're too tired to walk for 30 minutes, stay in bed and do a bit of Schumann, therapeutic blanket or chi machine. You have to accept this discomfort and the fact that you are very tired. Some people are not tired. Everyone is different. Strong symptoms are a positive sign of an elimination crisis. A fever is always beneficial because the immune system is maturing and cleansing toxins. Never stop a fever with chemical remedies.
6. Put some awareness into your dry fast, into your daily actions and into the words you use with others.
7. Incorporate yoga as much as possible, as it will help to detoxify and calm the nervous system.
8. Limit your words to what is strictly necessary: workshops and small talk. Don't talk if you're tired. Save your words for the end of the dry fast.
9. Incorporate notions of Prana into your breathing and use mental imagery and the breath to recharge your vital energy.
10. Save your energy for detoxification and renewal.
11. Avoid long calls with your loved ones, which will tire you out. Keep messages on WhatsApp to a minimum.
12. Have little contact with plant oils, except perhaps certain essential oils for inhalation, such as lavender or petit grain bigaradier.
13. Do not treat each other during the cure if you are a therapist. This will draw on your vital energy.
14. Depending on what the hotel or gîte has to offer, put a bottle or two of cold water at less than 11 degrees on your head or body if you feel any pain. This is optional.
15. Walk for at least 30 minutes a day, close to the hotel or in the surrounding area.
16. Do not put anything in your mouth, no mouthwash or toothpaste. You can use a tongue scraper. But wipe it dry when you apply it.

17. You are free to take part in the workshops or not. But remember to let me know on the Whatsapp group or on my phone, because if I don't see you in the morning, we'll automatically come and see you to check that everything's OK.
18. Kidney, liver and stomach symptoms are normal during dry fasting.
19. In the event of an emergency or accident, call 124 for an ambulance in Montenegro, 144 in Switzerland and 112 in Spain.
20. Take it easy when moving around to avoid dizziness. If you feel unwell, press one point right under your nose and apply peppermint essential oil or breathe in a little.
21. Don't go far on your own; it's better to go in pairs at least.
22. A little honey may be given to bring the sugar levels back up and the person may come out of the coma, but I have never seen this.
23. If someone is having too much trouble without water and the parameters are good, they can talk to me about it and I might be able to suggest that they come out of the fast with a small amount of water.
24. If the desire to drink becomes unbearable, first drink lukewarm or temperate water, in small sips, gradually. Never drink iced water or juice after a dry fast.
25. Do cardiac coherence at least three times five minutes a day, it will calm your heart and oxygenate you. Do this as much as possible.
26. Use the massage ring to stimulate your body.
27. Do the Schumann plate every day for at least five minutes in each position.
28. If you feel like it, take advantage of the treatments on offer: massage, Ito thermie, etc.
29. Anchor in your body and your cells that all will be well and that your body is cleansing and regenerating itself.
30. 30. During this retreat, imagine yourself at the age of 20 and in great shape.

31. Don't take any personal initiative of any kind. Ask us before you do anything stupid.
32. Although the nights during dry fasting can be long, try to go to bed early, remembering that even if you lie down without sleeping, you will also recover energy. Regular waking at night is normal.
33. The safety check is as follows: if your pulse is at +110 for more than two hours, or you have high blood pressure for more than two hours with readings of more than 160 and 100, this is a sign that you should stop the dry fast. If tiredness and lack of vital energy prevent you from walking for at least five minutes, or if you feel very dizzy, you can decide yourself to stop fasting. Let me know in any case. I can also ask you to stop dry fasting.
34. If there is no weight loss over 48 hours, this is abnormal. This indicates intoxication and the need to start drinking water again.
35. If you don't have any urine for 24 hours, that's no good either and you need to refeed and take the water and broth again. If no urine comes out in 24 hours, please tell me about it.
36. The weight loss threshold is 45%, so a person weighing 100kg should not lose less than 55kg.
37. The bar at heart level is abnormal; it also signals the end of dry fasting and the resumption of water and then soups rapidly.
38. The three progressive dry fasting cures are: a short detox of three to five days, an annual maintenance cure with a well-being detox of five to seven days, and a cure of seven to nine days of dry fasting for a complete renewal of the body and treatment of pathologies. Three cures a year is ideal if you suffer from a chronic pathology. Follow up with a maintenance cure once a year.
39. You should never force yourself during your dry fast; go for it with heart and gentleness. Practise the whirling dervish, if you feel like it.

40. Dry fasting with no subsequent changes is a waste of time, just an experiment.
41. The key to success is to make the dietary and lifestyle changes that follow the cure and to change things in your life.
42. Use the food combinations recommended above.
43. Avoid too much mental activity during the dry fast as this consumes too much energy. The cure is not a place where you need to store up knowledge, but rather an inner experience to introspect and find peace within yourself.
44. Too much physical activity will drain your energy. Avoid walking three to four hours a day, that's too much.
45. Don't worry if you see other fasters looking unwell and exhausted. It's normal to be exhausted with a drawn face.
46. A certain state of euphoria can occur during dry fasting. Be vigilant. Channel and welcome everything that happens to you without expending your energy unnecessarily.
47. Cellular elimination, excretion, waste evacuation and renewal are the key mechanisms of dry fasting.
48. The symptoms that we are trying to suppress during dry fasting suppress the effects and effectiveness of the young person. You have to leave it alone. The example of honey in fasting and hiking cures that I have seen is nonsense. If there is discomfort, you have to leave it to the body unless it is outside the acceptable norm.
49. As soon as you wake up, go for a walk and soak up the sun's energy. Take the melatonin from the light, but avoid sunbathing for too long.
50. There is a metabolic slowdown in dry fasting, so go about your day slowly without rushing; it's normal to be slow.
51. Be free in your programme of activities because following them excessively can block the letting go and the letting be.
52. As well as cardiac coherence, practise square breathing, kapalabhati and whirling dervish.

3. General contraindications to dry fasting

1. Vitality too low on a scale of one to ten, i.e. less than three. Mandatory consultation with the fast companion to assess your ability to undergo a dry fast. The Metatron device provides a precise assessment of your health and already gives an accurate opinion of your general state of health.
2. Malignant tumours and haemoblastosis (stages III to IV, particularly after the use of chemotherapy)
3. Active pulmonary tuberculosis
4. Taking an anti-depressant such as Prozac
5. Heavy drug and alcohol use
6. Acute and chronic active hepatitis
7. Cirrhosis of the liver, purulent inflammatory diseases of the respiratory and abdominal cavities
8. Stage 2 and 3 circulatory insufficiency
9. Insufficient heart rhythm and conduction or heart problems
10. Thrombophlebitis and thrombosis
11. Pregnancy and breast-feeding
12. Children under seven and people over 80, but this depends on the person's vitality
13. Type 1 diabetes
14. Neurotic patients on medication

4. Fasting and medication

Medication should be avoided during fasting, but in some cases this is not possible. You should therefore take your medication if you experience too many symptoms, with or without water if possible. Dosages should be reduced because fasting makes you much more sensitive and the drugs have a greater effect because there is no food to act as a buffer. Before dry fasting, it is important to tell us if you are taking any of the following medicines, which require the greatest attention:

- steroid, cortisone
- non-steroidal anti-inflammatory drugs (NSAIDs)
- anti-hypertensive drugs (particularly Prozac, beta blockers and diuretics)
- oral antidiabetics and insulin
- contraceptive pill (sometimes with limited effects)
- anticoagulant
- psychotropic drugs (particularly neuroleptics and lithium)
- Antiepileptics

5. Is your immune system in good health?

A healthy immune system is essential to protect you against common illnesses such as colds and flu. When these infections become epidemic and you find yourself frequently ill, this may indicate a deficiency in your immune system. This triggers the body to look for ways to compensate, for example by developing a cold, which has been identified as "programmed immunity shutdown".

Frequent disorders can also signal a highly intoxicated body, filled with debris such as dead cell particles and excess protein, clogging up intercellular spaces and sometimes saturating lymphatic vessels. This accumulation of 'junk' impedes the body's optimal functioning, disrupting cellular communication and reducing the strength of electrical signals between cells, making the body more vulnerable to infection.

The intestine plays a crucial role in the health of your immune system. A porous gut can weaken immunity and affect your mental state, as diet and exercise have a direct impact on immune function, as does exposure to toxic emotional environments.

As a result, an organism clogged with waste becomes a hospitable host for a variety of bacteria and viruses. These pathogens feed on dead and contaminated cells, transforming them into liquid waste which is then eliminated by the lymphatic and blood systems towards the kidneys and other excretion routes. In short, by admitting its inability to clean itself, the body ends up resorting to bacteria and viruses to purify itself, particularly those already present in small quantities in the body or those contracted from outside.

To strengthen your immune system, it is therefore crucial to adopt a healthy lifestyle, including a balanced diet rich in nutrients, regular physical exercise and reducing exposure to negative emotional stress. Taking care of your body and mind is the key to maintaining a robust immune system ready to fight disease.

6. Encourage detox at all costs

The concept of illness, according to Dr Hammer's innovative vision and the new medicine, is to be interpreted not as a plague but as a saving manifestation, a protective mechanism that the body deploys to defend itself. Every symptom carries a message, an invitation to understand and cooperate rather than fight. The traditional approach to medicine, which is based on combating disease primarily with drugs produced by a flourishing pharmaceutical industry, is often criticised for failing to tackle the root causes of the problem. Indeed, Dr A. Zalmanov has already denounced this "pharmaceutical bacchanal", a trend that shows no sign of slowing down.

Unfortunately, the human body, particularly in the modern context of unsuitable eating habits and a sedentary lifestyle, has difficulty in effectively eliminating waste and dead cells. This slowness in the natural detoxification process highlights the importance of adopting practices such as dry fasting, recommended at least twice a year, to boost the body's self-cleansing capacities.

Infections and illnesses are often wrongly perceived as enemies to be eradicated. However, they can be seen as helpers, a kind of nurse who helps to cleanse the body of its internal waste products, which cannot otherwise be eliminated. This perspective is supported by the idea that the symptoms of immunodeficiency appear to allow our beneficial microflora to work more effectively during periods of illness.

So, fighting microbes seems to be an inadequate response to a society that does not recognise the usefulness of these agents in the natural healing process. Illness, often temporarily suppressed by conventional treatments, can return in a more severe form. This is why it is crucial to embrace the pillars of health, such as diet, exercise and lifestyle, to allow the body to experience a saving crisis, an exacerbation necessary for healing.

Dry fasting appears to be a profoundly purifying method, encouraging self-digestion (autolysis) of cellular debris and superfluous proteins. This natural detoxification process reduces the need for intervention by microbes and viruses, allowing the body to restore its balance and strengthen its immune defences. During fasting, a beneficial change in the intestinal microflora also occurs, similar to that observed in centenarians and yogis, improving the synthesis of biologically active and essential substances such as amino acids and enzymes.

In conclusion, illness should be seen not as an enemy but as an ally, a signal that our body is sending us to indicate the need for change. By adopting a holistic approach and cooperating with our body through healthy eating, dry fasting and an active lifestyle, we can facilitate a natural and sustainable healing process. This requires a paradigm shift, where true healing begins with a deep and respectful understanding of our body's signals.

CHAPTER 13

General mechanisms and symptoms of dry fasting

1. Symptoms during fasting

- **Elimination attacks or worsening of symptoms**

Dry fasting works in order of priority. The following symptoms can generally signal a curative crisis: fever, migraine, vomiting, acidosis, biliary or renal colic, cardiac disorder, arrhythmia, infectious disease, reddening of the skin, painful scars or flare-ups of an old pathology.

- **Weakness and fatigue**

It's normal because detox makes you tired in order to eliminate. If you feel better, there is less detox to do. Weakness is generally assessed on a scale of one to ten several times during the cure. Depending on this and your personal impression, too little vitality is a sign that your body no longer has enough energy to do the work of cleansing and renewal. It's common to feel a certain weakness during a fast, and it's important to be prepared for this. Often by the second day fatigue begins to set in and there may be times when even getting out of bed becomes difficult. However, this should not be a cause for concern.

General weakness accompanied by drowsiness and a lack of motivation to move indicates an energy deficit. You can regenerate your energy resources with cold-water affusions, yoga, meditation, gentle massages, the Schumann plateau and barefoot walks. In summer, exposure to the sun for 30 minutes a day is particularly beneficial.

The effectiveness of these methods is increased tenfold when you are in deep contact with nature. A spiritual connection with the natural elements is always beneficial: inwardly greeting the Earth with gratitude. By feeling this harmony and mutual understanding, we can perceive the response of the elements to our salvation.

When you're feeling very tired, it's a good idea to lie down and rest in the regenerative savasana yoga position. However, it is not advisable to lie down for too long. After a rest, a walk in the fresh air is recommended to feel invigorated. Generally speaking, after a difficult period comes relief and a desire to move, walk and communicate. Many people remain in excellent spirits right up to the end of their dry fast.

- **Nausea, regurgitation and vomiting during dry fasting**

When you feel weak and unwell and want to stop fasting, get moving, walk and do yoga. Gentle physical activity and gentle massages or yoga during fasting work all the organs and muscles. It gets the blood circulating and speeds up the cleansing process. Apathy is not as strong and passes more quickly after an hour's walk. On the contrary, giving in to apathy reinforces it and prolongs the body's cleansing process. Bear in mind that the body needs three times as much fresh air during fasting. So, take a walk or stay in the fresh air.

People with digestive problems often experience acid regurgitation during their first fasts. When such regurgitation occurs, the stomach has not been sufficiently cleansed. In the most serious cases, when regurgitation is aggravated by persistent heartburn and two to three daily cleansings do not give the desired result, you can drink small quantities of still mineral water diluted with added sorbents such as Silicea med.

Green or even black vomiting may occur if the liver is diseased. Vomiting is a sign that the liver is beginning to clear, the general condition may worsen and irritation may increase, which may mean that the dry fast is stopped if there is too much vomiting. It is safer to simply wait several days. You can also wash the stomach with hot or even very hot water and apply a hot water bottle to the liver.

- **Dizziness and blurred vision**

When you suddenly stand up, the blood can be redistributed rapidly, concentrating in the abdomen and leaving the head with insufficient blood supply. This can cause dizziness. Although there is generally no serious danger, apart from the risk of falling or hitting an object, it is advisable to take a few moments to sit on the edge of the bed before getting up or moving around.

Dizziness can also be linked to liver overload, requiring drainage or regeneration of the liver before starting a course of treatment. They often occur after standing up quickly, which is described as a gravitational or orthostatic collapse. The resulting sensation of blurred vision usually dissipates within a few seconds, but it is important to note that the person may fall during this time without losing consciousness entirely. This is due to an abrupt redistribution of blood, the volume of which tends to diminish during fasting. To avoid any complications, it is best to stand up slowly, using a support such as the back of a chair or a wall, especially after a hot bath in the bathroom.

Blurred vision is a symptom more frequently observed and particularly pronounced in tall, slim people. On the other hand, those who maintain regular outdoor activity, avoid being bedridden for too long and keep themselves occupied with exciting activities, are generally less likely to experience these inconveniences.

- **Fever**

A fever may occur during dry fasting. A fever is beneficial because it shows that your immune system is working to eliminate toxins and toxic products. In principle, you should never break a fever. Rest and wait for it to pass.

- **Headaches**

Headaches indicate increased detoxification and acidification of ketone bodies. They indicate that the blood is heavily contaminated. Headaches usually appear before the acidosis attack. Care should be taken in confined spaces or inside a vehicle, when toxins cannot be eliminated by breathing.

Headaches disappear if we help the oxygen to burn and the waste disposal systems to eliminate waste. So it's best to take more gentle walks and rest. If, however, the headaches are unbearable, you can use peppermint as an olfactory agent and add some to the temples. If, however, the headaches continue, you need to get out of the dry fast and make a good recovery while working on your liver and intestines.

- **Stomach aches**

They are often linked to the release of gas and can even occur after ten days of dry fasting. Bile production varies, which can cause vomiting, spasms and acid reflux. These discomforts can also be linked to emotional upsets.

Tummy massages, Schumann plate massages and treatments, full-body massages or ito thermie can soothe them, as can hot or cold water bottles. Flower field mattresses can also soothe any pain. At the start of fasting, acid secretions from the stomach are not buffered by food. They can therefore irritate the gastric mucosa.

- **The desire to eat**

Fighting the feeling of hunger is not so difficult to manage. You have to try to avoid thinking too much about eating and food. This can be done more easily by concentrating on inner work. You need to have a clear state of mind about what you want in your life. Say to yourself "I have nothing to eat and nothing to compensate for, that's just the way it is" and your subconscious will know that this is not a deception, so hunger won't cause too many problems.

From days 2 and 3, the feeling of hunger disappears completely, and the sight and smell of food no longer provoke salivation. It's more the water that can provoke cravings, especially if it's hot. However, it can happen that the fasting person is constantly thinking about food and anticipating the pleasure of feasting after the fast has been broken. You really mustn't go into this and return to your inner self, while asking for help from the person accompanying you on a dry fast.

However, it is necessary to bear in mind that the feeding centre in the brain is reflexively excited by any contact with and sight of food, especially in those who are new to fasting. This strongly interferes with the proper activation of the internal feeding mechanism. Those who are fasting should refrain from preparing food and avoid being present at other people's meals. Failure to do so often leads to sleep disturbances, headaches, heartburn and irritation.

- **Smelly breath**

On the third day of fasting, an unpleasant odour may emanate from the breath, especially if the body has not undergone sufficient purification. This odour is attributed to the release of insufficiently oxidised compounds, with the predominant scent often reminiscent of acetone. However, putrid, malodorous odours and other equally 'charming' scents can sometimes mingle. For those fasting to the point of an attack for the first time, the breath can become so nauseating that it can be difficult to stay in the same room as the person. One can only imagine the abundance of toxins and waste that person has had in their body!

As the body undergoes the purification process, the intensity of the smell gradually diminishes and by the seventh day it subsides. It is crucial to help the lungs expel as many toxins as possible during this period. Recommended methods include yoga, regular walks, ice water affusions and breathing.

- **Tachycardia**

Your heart function enables the blood to supply your cells with oxygen and glucose, and to expel waste products. It reflects what your body is going through. Under the influence of the "sympathetic" nervous system and the intense work of elimination, the heartbeat speeds up. The loss of minerals can also explain this tachycardia. There is a mudra that protects and calms, as well as su jok points on the hand.

- **Hridaya Mudra**

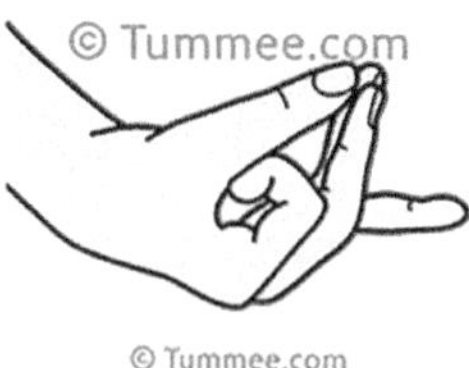

Hridaya Mudra, also known as Heart Mudra, is a hand position used in yoga practice to help calm the mind and balance the emotions. Here's how to perform the Hridaya Mudra with one or two hands:

Hridaya Mudra with one hand:

1. Sit comfortably with your back straight.
2. Open the palm of your right or left hand.
3. Bend your index finger so that it touches the base of your thumb.
4. Bring the tip of the thumb to touch the tip of the middle and ring fingers while the little finger remains extended.
5. Place the hand with the mudra on your knee or in your lap, palm upwards.
6. Breathe calmly and concentrate on your heart or breathing.

- **Hridaya Mudra with two hands**

1. Repeat the same steps as above for each hand.
2. Place both hands in Hridaya Mudra on your lap or in your lap, palms upwards.
3. Breathe calmly and concentrate on your heart or breathing.

   Hridaya Mudra is often used to promote relaxation and inner peace. It is said to help open the heart chakra and release blocked emotions. Practise this mudra for a few minutes each day to feel the benefits.

- **Benefits for physical and mental health. Here are the main benefits of practising this mudra regularly**

1. **Calming stress and anxiety.** The Hridaya Mudra helps to calm the mind and reduce stress and anxiety. It promotes a feeling of peace and tranquillity.
2. **Improving heart health.** This mudra is thought to benefit the heart by regulating blood circulation and stabilising the heartbeat.
3. **Emotional balancing.** It helps to balance the emotions, reducing feelings of anger and sadness. It is often used to open the heart chakra and release blocked emotions.
4. **Relief from depression.** Regular practice of Hridaya Mudra can help to alleviate the symptoms of depression.
5. **Improved breathing.** By helping to relax the body and mind, this mudra can also improve the quality of breathing.
6. **Reducing blood pressure.** Thanks to its calming effects, the Hridaya Mudra can help to lower high blood pressure.
7. **Strengthening the inner connection.** This mudra promotes greater self-awareness and a deeper connection with the heart and inner emotions.
8. **Improves concentration and meditation.** It is useful for deepening meditation practice and improving concentration.

9. **Support during convalescence**. Hridaya Mudra can be beneficial for those recovering from heart disease or other illnesses, supporting the healing process.
   It is important to practise this mudra in a calm and comfortable environment, and to concentrate on breathing deeply and regularly to maximise the benefits. As with any yoga or meditation practice, it is advisable to consult a health professional or qualified instructor if in doubt or if you have a specific medical condition.

- **Urine darkens considerably during dry fasting**

They become loaded with urea and ammonia, bile pigments and phosphate. They become dark, odorous and abundant during the first few days of fasting, but this can continue. The more colourful and odorous they are, the greater the number of toxins to be eliminated. No urination during a fast indicates a kidney problem that you should address immediately, by hydrating with nettle tea and taking broths. Your kidneys also need rest to regenerate. Dry fasting forces your body to take water from your tissues and fat so that your kidneys can function. If you do not urinate, it is essential to break your dry fast.

- **Pain and the return of old illnesses**

The increase in pain is linked to a momentary worsening of inflammation on the second and third day of fasting. This is due to the over-production of cortisol, like a return of old illnesses that have not been completely cured. Keep your spirits up; this is not a regression, but a chance to put an end to it once and for all.

- **The white tongue**

It is linked to the slowing down of your intestine. Toxins pass through the walls of the intestine, from the external environment (mouth to anus) to the internal environment (blood, hormones). As the lungs are also an emunctory, your tongue ends up loaded with toxins and turns very white. Your breath becomes stronger, especially as the ketone bodies you produce include acetone.

- **Heavy sweat**

It is concentrated in mineral salts, which makes it more fragrant. Entering the room of a fasting person is like entering the room of a garlic eater.

You may feel hot or cold. The lack of calories ingested and the drop in thyroid hormone secretion to allow energy use to be reduced can cause a sensation of cold. A sensation of heat reflects a great deal of elimination work, but generally after four or five days, the heat intensifies in dry fasting.

Cramps. These are linked to the loss of potassium and calcium at the start of fasting. The muscles can no longer relax.

- **Back pain**

The hinge joint that connects the pelvis to the lumbar vertebrae is subject to a great deal of stress. The older we get, because of acidity and wear, the more a general degenerative process sets in. Back muscle tension may appear in the first few days of dry fasting. The elimination of water can cause a slight mineral imbalance and changes in the hydration of the intervertebral discs. Physiologically, the metabolism becomes more acidic during dry fasting, which can also contribute to lower back pain. Locally applied heat can relieve this pain.

- **Eyesight can deteriorate after dry fasting**

Blurred vision and vertigo often occur after a sudden rise from a sitting or lying position: this is called gravitational or orthostatic collapse. A few seconds later, the sensation of blurred vision usually passes, but the person may fall during this time, although the loss of consciousness is not usually total.

This condition is caused by a sudden redistribution of blood, the volume of which decreases during fasting. There is no danger in this, but it is best to stand up slowly, holding onto the back of a chair or a wall (especially in the bathroom after a hot bath).

Blurred vision is most often encountered and most clearly pronounced in tall, thin people. Visual acuity may be reduced during dry fasting and even for weeks afterwards, but all will return to normal with an improvement in vision. This phenomenon is temporary and is probably due to a reduction in intraocular pressure, which modifies the curvature of the crystalline lens.

- **Dry mouth**

Given the temporary lack of water, this can lead to an imbalance in mineral resources, especially in the case of a reduction in potassium, which is abundant in saliva.

- **Hypoglycaemia**

During a dry fast, you need to move but not force yourself, so as to stimulate your emunctories while avoiding violent efforts that require too much sugar. Gentle, conscious walking, yoga, massages and the Schumann plate mobilise the joints and muscles. Dry fasters who engage in too much physical activity expose themselves to hypoglycaemia. This will manifest itself as severe fatigue after exercise and muscle soreness. Remedy: take the three rests.

- **Pain during dry fasting**

In dry fasting, the appearance of symptoms and pain is quite frequent. This is a sign of real therapeutic work going on inside the body. In juice diets and water fasts, this work is less present and there is little reaction or pain in the body. The pain experienced during fasting can be frightening but should be experienced as an integral part of the healing and cleansing process. This pain often reflects the repair of damaged tissue and the cleansing of the body. These symptoms usually disappear quickly after release, although in some cases they may return. As each person is unique, the renovation process and the order of healing vary from one individual to another, but it is often the most important problems that are treated first. Sometimes, unexpected pain can occur, signalling the prevention of as yet undetected illnesses, such as unexplained pain in a joint that may indicate the onset of arthritis.

Extreme cases, such as severe headaches, may require interventions such as several consecutive enemas after fasting and the use of sorbents to relieve the pain. Acute pain can also occur when kidney stones pass. Hot baths and sauna sessions can help. However, sometimes the stones dissolve and disappear without causing any noticeable pain.

It is important to understand that these symptoms are temporary and are part of the body's natural process of purification and restructuring during and after dry fasting.

- **Fasting and impatience in the legs**

This unpleasant sensation, which generally occurs at night and when lying down, can be relieved by taking cold showers, using the Schumann tray, the "Champs des fleurs" mat or rubbing with organic essential oils.

- **Skin rashes**

Sometimes associated with itching, redness and acne may appear locally. This is detoxification and the waste products leave the skin. The skin may be irritated by perspiration laden with toxins and acids released during fasting. It is also possible that stored waste or traces of medication in the fat are relegated to the skin.

- **Sleep disturbances**

The desire to sleep disappears during fasting. If this does not cause serious discomfort, you can stay awake for as long as you like. Sleep can be severely disrupted during dry fasting, and even more so in people who are highly intoxicated. However, sleep disturbances do not mean that fasting is not indicated. On the contrary, once properly detoxified, some people can improve their sleep because renovations have been made throughout the body, including the central nervous system. I always say in my retreats that you shouldn't necessarily go for a walk at night, but rather try to stay in bed, because despite everything, we recover energy during the night. Never forget that it's at night that we repair ourselves and that detoxification is at its strongest. As soon as you've had your water, food and protein, you'll be back asleep in no time. It should also be noted that as long as we sleep badly, there is toxaemia and a probable latent pathology. If sleep improves over the days, which is rare, this means that the toxins have been expelled and there is no need to go too far with dry fasting. If the inability to sleep disturbs you, then after four to five days of insomnia, once you are exhausted, use the usual methods: daily walks and cold affusions. Fasting should be stopped and repeated in two or three months. A specialist consultation is necessary.

2. How dry fasting takes care of your ailments

In addition to its preventive effects and its ability to facilitate the elimination of waste and toxins and rejuvenate the body, therapeutic dry fasting also helps to relax the central nervous system. The practice is likened to peeling an onion, with each layer representing a different stage of recovery. The healing process takes place in successive stages, and the effectiveness of these stages is directly influenced by the quality and regularity of the fasting sequences, as well as by the individual's lifestyle. A balanced diet, adequate hydration and restful sleep are all key elements that accompany fasting to optimise the health benefits.

The duration of the fast is a crucial factor. While short fasts can bring immediate benefits, the complete resolution of chronic and long-standing problems may require longer dry fasts, generally between six and ten days. In some cases, several cycles of fasting may be necessary to achieve complete healing. These prolonged periods of fasting allow deep detoxification and offer the body the opportunity to regenerate and repair itself more fully. The time between cures is also important, because if you leave more than six months between two cures, there will be little cumulative effect. The best results I've seen are with sessions every three months, with an average of four cures a year. But each case is different and needs to be analysed individually.

In conclusion, therapeutic dry fasting is a holistic approach to health, which respects the principles of Hering's Law. By treating health problems in order of urgency and reversing the course of time, this ancient practice promises a profound revitalisation of the body.

3. Link between vital force and toxaemia

However, our well-being is compromised when toxaemia prevails over vital force. Toxaemia, the accumulation of waste and toxins in the body, can overload our system, leaving it unable to function properly. To counter this overload, three types of rest are essential: physical, mental and digestive. These forms of rest facilitate the elimination of toxins, particularly when combined with gentle activities such as walking and specific biotherapies, which are often incorporated into our dry fasting cures.

Before starting a course of treatment, the main objective is to increase energy levels, in particular by improving mitochondrial function, in order to optimise the detoxification and cell renewal process. Certain techniques and food supplements may be recommended. Preparing for a cure also involves reducing toxins, so as to further enhance the benefits of dry fasting and prevent elimination crises. These crises occur when the body is overwhelmed by an excess of toxins that it can no longer manage effectively. They can occur even in slim individuals, where the more subtle toxins are linked to over-stimulation of the nervous system, hindering their elimination by somatic and nervous means.

It is crucial to recognise that the waste accumulated in our bodies may be endogenous, produced by our own metabolic processes, or exogenous, originating from environmental pollutants. Dry fasting is proving to be one of the most effective methods of reducing the toxic load while revitalising the vital force. It is essential to adopt an optimal lifestyle before and after fasting in order to maximise its benefits.

Incorporating practices such as meditation, yoga, ito termie, gentle massage or the pucma blanket can be beneficial in strengthening the mind-body connection, increasing the resilience of our nervous system to environmental and internal stresses. These practices promote a state of deep relaxation, allowing our bodies to regenerate and repair themselves more effectively, while improving the flow of prana or chi through our bodily systems. By cultivating presence and conscious attention, we become more able to perceive our body's subtle signals, guiding us towards the care it needs to maintain or regain its balance.

At the same time, the adoption of a nutrient-rich, balanced diet is necessary, as is the regular practice of dry fasting as a method of reducing toxaemia.

4. How do the emunctory organs work during dry fasting and how do they regenerate?

- **The liver.**

The liver, a central organ in the management of our health and well-being, plays a crucial role during fasting and benefits greatly from this practice for its regeneration. With more than 500 vital functions, including filtering the blood, storing vitamins and minerals and secreting bile, the liver is essential for detoxifying the body, eliminating toxins and purifying the blood.

During dry fasting, the liver takes advantage of a pause in the digestive process, allowing it to carry out a major internal 'housecleaning'. This period of rest facilitates autolysis, where the most damaged and toxic tissues are destroyed and eliminated. In this way, the liver repairs itself from within and regains its vitality and efficiency. The longer the fast, the more profound the repair. Dry fasting also reduces the amount of toxins entering the digestive tract, which relieves the liver and allows it to resume its normal functions in a healthier environment.

Fasting also encourages the liver to eliminate the overload of toxins that clog it up, promoting cleansing, repair and regeneration. The process of autolysis, or autophagy, plays a vital role here, selectively targeting damaged cells and tissues to break them down, enabling the liver to cleanse and revitalise itself.

Studies and observations on the impact of dry fasting on the liver, carried out with a scanner, reveal an improvement in liver function, with a reduction in the accumulation of fats in the liver, thus helping to prevent or reduce the risk of diseases such as cirrhosis. In addition, dry fasting has shown benefits in stimulating the production of enzymes beneficial to the liver, promoting better lipid metabolism and more effective regulation of blood glucose levels.

To optimise the benefits of dry fasting for the liver, it is advisable to prepare the body, and especially the liver, with the food preparation suggested in this book, by lightening the diet before the start of the fast. During dry fasting, it is also important to support the liver through exercises and biotherapies that do not take energy away from the body. This information underlines the importance of the liver to our overall health and highlights the potential benefits of dry fasting as a method of regenerating and strengthening this vital organ.

- **Kidneys**

Dry fasting is renowned for its many potential health benefits, including on kidney function. You can consult the recommended clinical studies at the beginning of the book. The absence of water intake forces the body to draw on its reserves, which could stimulate various physiological mechanisms and contribute to the regeneration and detoxification of the kidneys. The kidneys play a crucial role during dry fasting, adjusting and optimising the body's water balance. Reducing fluid intake could reduce the workload on the kidneys, allowing them to rest and regenerate. This process is thought to promote the repair of damaged kidney tissue and improve renal function. One notable effect of dry fasting is the increased concentration of urine resulting from the reduction in water intake. This increased concentration loads the urine with solids and waste products, facilitating their elimination and helping to cleanse the kidneys and urinary system of various accumulated waste products. Urinary infections and inflammations such as nephritis, cystitis and urethritis could also be affected by dry fasting. The argument is that the absence of water limits the environment necessary for the proliferation of infectious agents, thereby helping to resolve the infection without resorting to antibiotics and their potential side-effects.

Dry fasting has also been suggested as a potentially effective method of treating kidney stones. Reducing fluid intake may help dissolve and eliminate kidney stones, although the precise mechanism requires scientific validation. Although dry fasting may offer potential benefits for the kidneys and urinary system, the importance of a cautious and supervised approach is crucial, particularly for individuals with pre-existing health problems or specific kidney pathologies. Dry fasting has benefits for renal health through tissue regeneration, detoxification, and treatment of urinary pathologies.

- **The lungs**

Dry fasting is a method of purification and regeneration, particularly for its beneficial effects on the lungs. It has a positive effect on lung function and on various bronchopulmonary pathologies such as asthma.

As excretory organs, the lungs play a vital role in expelling the carbon dioxide formed during cellular metabolism. During dry fasting, metabolism slows down due to the reduced oxidation of carbons, thus modifying respiratory exchanges. Although breathing may become more superficial, the ability to expel mucus remains, contributing to the detoxification process.

One of the notable observations during dry fasting is the intensification of breath odour, a sign that the body is actively eliminating waste via the respiratory tract. In some particularly intoxicated people, this phenomenon can be so pronounced that it impairs the ability to breathe freely, indicating a massive elimination of toxins via the lungs.

It is crucial to understand that symptoms such as tonsillitis, rhinitis and sinusitis should not be artificially suppressed. These elimination processes are natural and necessary for the body, preventing the retention of toxins which, if artificially suppressed, could be redirected to other organs, creating further disorders.

Dry fasting offers the body a chance to purify itself and fight infections naturally, without the intervention of drugs that could mask symptoms or make the situation worse. This natural approach can be particularly effective in treating conditions such as pneumonia or bronchitis, often with noticeable improvements in just a few days.

- **The intestine**

Although the exact mechanisms by which the benefits of dry fasting modify the intestinal microbiome have not been precisely studied, it is clear that fasting induces positive changes. For example, studies on dry fasting in Russia, carried out by Professor Romanov, have shown a reversible change in the nature of intestinal bacteria, with a reduction in pathogenic germs and an increase in beneficial strains. This is the famous multiplication of stem cells that will regenerate the entire digestive mucosa. These adjustments also testify to the positive action of dry fasting on the well-being of the intestinal flora, effects that persist several months after the end of fasting.

The development of leaky gut or intestinal porosity is very well treated by dry fasting. This syndrome affects virtually everyone at some point in their lives, as a result of poor diet, excessive stress or illness. Normally, this problem resolves itself when conditions return to normal, but it can persist if the triggering factors remain.

Characterised by excessive inflammation caused by chronic activation of the immune system, leaky gut can give rise to a wide range of symptoms, from skin inflammation, joint pain and cognitive problems to classic digestive problems such as bloating, gas, constipation and/or diarrhoea. To recover from a leaky gut, it is crucial to restore the integrity of the digestive barriers, which can be achieved rapidly by dry fasting. By abstaining from all food and emptying the digestive system for several days, the presence of agents that degrade the intestinal barrier and the intestinal microbiota, such as food particles and toxic chemicals, is considerably reduced. This allows the digestive system to regenerate rapidly in a calmer immune environment. Combining dry fasting with stress-reduction techniques and the use of certain herbs and dietary supplements such as fir resin or zeolite can amplify the healing effect.

If left untreated, intestinal porosity can persist for a long time and set the stage for the development of more serious intestinal health problems, inflammation-based diseases or cancers. However, it can be relatively easy to treat when the right steps are taken. We also understand that in the absence of food, the digestive system is no longer called upon to digest, and can concentrate on detoxifying and repairing itself through the process of autolysis, where cells regenerate and rid themselves of toxins. This internal cleansing promotes a rebalancing of the microbiota, with healthy strains adapting to a new homeostatic balance. Intermittent fasting has also demonstrated positive effects on the richness of the microbiota, suggesting that even short periods of food abstinence can encourage the renewal and enrichment of the intestinal flora.

These findings underline the importance of dry fasting not only as a tool for revitalising the body, but also as a means of supporting and improving digestive and overall health. The benefits observed for the intestinal microbiota, such as reduced inflammation and the promotion of beneficial flora, contribute to better overall health. However, it is crucial to note that these studies, although promising, are often based on small cohorts and that more research is needed to confirm these effects and better understand the mechanisms involved. Despite this, the current results offer an interesting perspective on the potential of dry fasting as a means of promoting optimal intestinal health and, by extension, a better quality of life. It's also important to understand that without water, the reorganisation process dries out certain germs such as candidiasis, Helicobacter pylori and even certain parasites much more quickly. Hydrating them will result in them proliferating again and again, hence the dual benefit of dry fasting, which will enable better regeneration thanks to stem cells and a reduction in pathogenic bacteria.

- **The skin**

The skin, an extensive and highly exposed organ, plays a crucial role in our equilibrium by providing a barrier against various aggressions, eliminating toxins thanks to its sweat and sebaceous glands, and helping to regulate body temperature. It also contributes to the synthesis of vitamin D and acts as a sensory interface with the environment. However, modern lifestyles can take their toll on the skin, accelerating its ageing process. Dry fasting is a beneficial way of counteracting these effects and revitalising the skin. In fact, during dry fasting, the body cleanses itself deeply through autolysis, allowing cells to regenerate and organs to purify. This process may induce temporary skin reactions, reflecting the purifying effect of fasting on the skin.

Skin health is essential for a number of reasons. It detoxifies, supports immunity and acts as a protective barrier. Unhealthy skin can reveal an internal imbalance, manifested by symptoms such as paleness, early wrinkles and acne. Adopting a healthier lifestyle, particularly with regard to diet, can help resolve these problems.

Dry fasting is the ultimate method for regenerating the skin and wrinkles. We have experience of seeing faces rejuvenated, but also of seeing skin conditions such as pimples improve dramatically. Digestive rest plays a significant role in skin health. It purifies the blood and eases the workload on the emunctories, enabling the skin to become healthier. Participants in a dry fasting course often notice an improvement in the appearance of their skin, with fewer imperfections and a more relaxed, rejuvenated appearance. This transformation is also supported by the release of feel-good hormones, such as serotonin and endorphins, as well as growth hormones and stem cells.

The experience of five to nine days of dry fasting offers visible benefits for the skin. A gradual approach, such as a mono-diet of vegetables, good fats or intermittent fasting, can be a good starting point for those wishing to explore the positive effects of dry fasting on their skin, without committing to a more intensive approach.

Ultimately, our skin is a reflection of our inner health and well-being. Taking care of your skin also means taking care of yourself. Dry fasting is an invaluable ally in this quest for well-being, helping to purify and regenerate our largest organ.

5. Increased heart rate during dry fasting

Dry fasting has a significant influence on various aspects of human physiology, particularly the heart rate. This phenomenon, often observed in the form of an accelerated pulse, or tachycardia, can be attributed to a number of physiological and metabolic factors.

6. Influence of the sympathetic nervous system

The sympathetic nervous system plays a key role in regulating heart rate. In response to dry fasting, this system can be activated to increase the heart rate. This reaction is part of the 'fight or flight' mechanism, preparing the body to cope with stressful or emergency situations. Fasting, by depriving the body of its usual supply of energy and water, can be interpreted as stress, leading to an increased heart rate.

7. Intense elimination work and loss of minerals

During dry fasting, the body intensifies its efforts to eliminate toxins and metabolic waste. This increased work of elimination requires more oxygen and nutrients, which leads to an increase in cardiac activity to satisfy its increased needs. The loss of minerals, particularly sodium and potassium, which can occur during dry fasting, also affects the heart rate. These minerals are essential for the transmission of electrical signals in the heart, and their imbalance can lead to tachycardia.

8. Cardiac variability and detoxification

Cardiac variability, which refers to variations in the time between heartbeats, is considered to be an indicator of heart health. Dry fasting can induce a higher variability, a sign of the body's increased capacity to adapt to different physiological stresses. During fasting, the detoxification process accelerates, requiring more intense cardiac activity to transport waste products out of the cells and excrete them efficiently.

Although increased heart rate and heart variability may play a role in detoxification and weight loss during dry fasting, it is crucial to monitor these changes to avoid negative health consequences. Persistent tachycardia, especially if it exceeds 110 beats per minute over a long period, may signal excessive stress on the heart and necessitate discontinuation of dry fasting.

It is also important to note that physiological reactions to dry fasting can vary considerably from one person to another. Factors such as general state of health, age and preparation for fasting influence how the body reacts.

In conclusion, although dry fasting can offer benefits in terms of detoxification and weight loss, it is essential to pay attention to the body's signals, particularly with regard to cardiac activity.

9. Observation of vitals during dry fasting

Dry fasting, which involves abstaining from food and water, requires you to pay close attention to the signals your body is sending out. Regular observation of certain physiological constants can help you to navigate this experience in a more informed and safe way. Here are the essential elements to monitor during this period.

- **State of Vitality**

Assess and record your energy levels and your state of vitality at different times of the day: morning, noon and evening. These observations can vary considerably from one day to the next. It is evaluated on a sheet of paper from one to ten. Vitality one means that you can't even get out of bed to walk 20 steps. Your state of tiredness is a determining factor during dry fasting and, according to the person accompanying you, if the vitality level is too low, the dry fasting will have to be stopped. It is quite normal to feel tired during dry fasting, as the elimination of toxins takes up a lot of the body's energy. Some dry fasters retain a great deal of energy during their fast, which is a very good sign as it is a sign of basic vitality, maintained by a healthy lifestyle. Although vitality returns fairly quickly as soon as food and water are resumed, some fasters experience persistent fatigue, which means that the dry fast has been cut short too quickly during intense detoxification.

This also means that dry fasting should be repeated, if possible, within the following 12 months. During dry fasting, it is crucial to practise relaxation, yoga, conscious walking, the Schuman plateau, gentle massage, meditation, cardiac coherence, the chi machine, the Pucma therapeutic blanket and ito termie. The aim of all these biotherapies will be to increase energy and relax the central nervous system, and that's all we want in order to have maximum energy to detoxify and renew your tissues and organs.

- **Weight**

Monitoring your weight is crucial. During dry fasting, weight loss is expected due to the absence of food and water intake and the consumption of fat and body reserves for energy. Make a note of your weight every morning to monitor this process. The safety weight is not really important, it's mainly vitality that we're looking at, but in general a loss of more than 45% of your starting weight could signal the need for a recovery, which still leaves us plenty of margin. When it comes to resuming eating, if the weight is low when you leave, you need to resume eating very slowly, gradually over a very long period.

- **Pulse**

Your pulse may reflect the intensity of the effort your body has to make to adapt to fasting. An increase in heart rate (tachycardia) may occur, due to the activation of the sympathetic nervous system and the intensified elimination of toxins. It is advisable to measure your pulse in the morning, at midday and in the evening. A pulse that is too high for too long is a sign that dry fasting has come to an end.

- **Urine**

Observing the colour, odour and viscosity of your urine can provide clues as to how intoxicated you are and how well your body is eliminating waste. Dark, smelly urine can indicate a high concentration of waste, as can pain on urination. After six days of dry fasting, leave a urine sample in a glass to observe the changes and you will see sediments that are called encrusted waste and that only dry fasting, by lymphatic drainage, can remove. Even a three-week water fast will not allow this encrusted waste to come out. This is clearly visible in the urine glass test.

- **Blood Pressure**

Taking your blood pressure is another key indicator of your health during dry fasting. Variations may occur due to changes in your blood volume and your body's adaptation to fasting. It is crucial never to exceed 20-30% of your usual blood pressure. Your fasting consultant will tell you whether you should stop dry fasting.

- **Tongue and breath**

The condition of your tongue (colour, coating) and the quality of your breath can also indicate your body's state of detoxification. A heavy tongue or strong breath can indicate active elimination of toxins from the lungs. You can draw the following conclusion: as long as there is waste coming out and a heavy tongue, the toxins are still there and a single fast will not be enough to eliminate them all. We can also look at a mouth chart to check where the marks are that mean certain organs are affected.

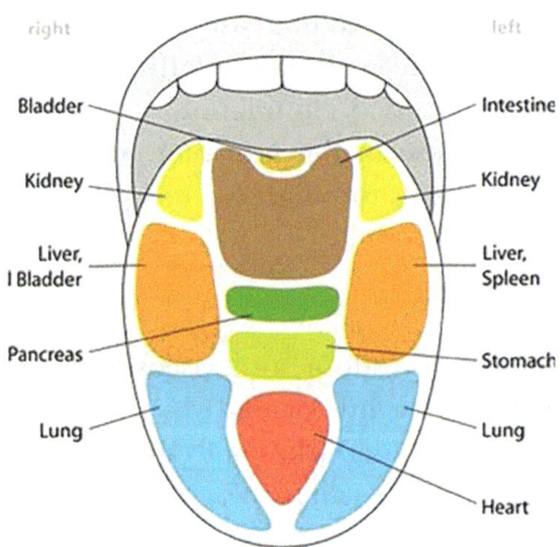

CHAPTER 14

The physiological effects of fasting

1. Restructuring and self-healing after dry fasting

Restructuring and self-healing are remarkable processes that occur during dry fasting, particularly when it is practised over a period of seven days or more. During this period, the liver plays a crucial role by intensifying the elimination of bile. This activity can lead to a change in the colour of the urine due to the increased presence of bilirubin. If the bile does not reach the kidneys properly, it can rise, causing vomiting, indicating a potentially overloaded liver and insufficient preparation for fasting. The liver, with its 400 or so vital functions, benefits from an opportunity to regenerate and renew itself thanks to this process.

The stomach too is subject to regeneration by autolysis, renewing and repairing itself for up to three weeks after the end of dry fasting. This regeneration also extends to the pancreas, offering promising prospects, even for difficult pathologies such as type 1 diabetes.

Improvements have also been seen in the skin, with a general improvement in the condition of the skin. General blood circulation and kidney function improve, as does prostate health. The respiratory tract, including the bronchi and lungs, also benefits from this process, suggesting a potential improvement in various bronchopulmonary pathologies. Finally, endocrine function, essential for the body's hormonal balance, is also likely to be repaired and improved.

2. The general therapeutic effects of dry fasting

2.1 Detoxification effects

When the body fasts, it tries to get rid of anything that consumes energy without providing any benefit. As a result, toxins stored in the body are excreted. Research has shown high levels of endorphins, the hormones that make us feel good and happy after fasting.

It has been shown that not eating for a single day improves the body's ability to detoxify toxins and keep other organs such as the liver and kidneys working properly.

2.2 Effects on DNA and the genome

A recent study shows the benefits of fasting, even for a short period, in improving DNA methylation. Other studies should be carried out to show that fasting can restore fragile genetics. Explorations should also be carried out on autistic diseases. https://clinicalepigeneticsjournal.biomedcentral.com/articles/10.1186/s13148-017-0340-8

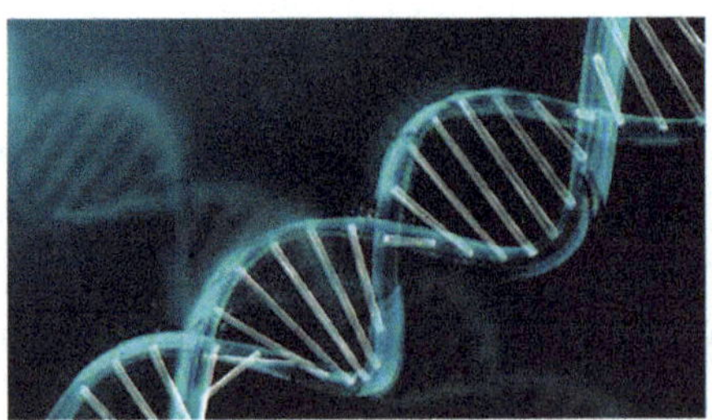

2.3 Effects on inflammation

Autoimmune diseases such as arthritis, polyarthritis, allergies, asthma or digestive diseases (colitis, gastritis) are successfully treated. Blood fat, sugar, uric acid and certain pathological structures and proteins are burnt in the metabolic fire in "autodigestion" or "autophagy" mode. This occurs thanks to the concomitant production of hormones such as glucagon or growth hormone STH, as well as a drop in insulin. Other excess substances can also be eliminated by stimulating kidney, intestinal and respiratory functions.

2.4 Effects on organs

On the liver:

- Elimination and neutralisation of toxins.
- Increase in HDL cholesterol levels.
- Lower total cholesterol and triglyceride levels.
- Lower LDL cholesterol.
- Total liver regeneration.

In 84% of cases, fasting improved the condition of people suffering from other serious illnesses, such as steatosis and hypercholesterolaemia. It also considerably reduced their fatigue. Fasting can also correct obesity if carried out at regular intervals and under controlled conditions. A useful note: 93% of the subjects studied did not feel hungry during the fast.

On the intestines:

Dry fasting improves the intestinal flora, the microbiota and the balance of the microbiota by balancing the bacteria. Excess bacteria are eliminated and the missing ones multiply! To promote good health, the return to food must be perfectly adapted, which is what will enable you to maintain a healthy flora over the long term.

For women, their vaginal flora depends on their intestinal flora. If the microbiota is healthy, so is the vaginal flora. Dry fasting also helps to regenerate the intestinal barrier.

On the brain:

- Greater protection for neurons against dysfunction and degeneration.
- Increase in BDNF factor
- Increased creation of new neurons.
- Increased brain plasticity
- Reduced neuronal excitotoxicity
- Increased levels of neurotrophins (BDNF), proteins that promote the regeneration and growth of neurons
- Significant increase in the secretion of somatotropin (growth hormone)
- Autophagy of dysfunctional or damaged cells
- Increase in ketones in the brain which reduce oxidative stress and glutamate
- Reduced inflammatory activity

Mark Mattson, a neuroscientist who has studied the ageing of the brain, considers fasting to be a weapon for preventing Alzheimer's disease, dementia and memory loss. Like sport, fasting induces the production of BDNF (brain-derived neurotrophic factor). These proteins have a dual effect: they increase the number of mitochondria, our body's energy generators, in nerve cells and produce new neurons in the hippocampus. They also help to improve mood. The production of BDNF is also accompanied by an increase in serotonin, known as the 'happy hormone'.

On the pancreas:

Regulation of blood sugar levels (50% reduction in glucose and insulin-like growth factor 1) and increased sensitivity to insulin.

Fasting could reduce your risk of developing diabetes. Research has shown that fasting just once a week, and drinking only water on that day, can reduce the risk of developing diabetes. Fasting also reduces cholesterol levels and blood pressure.

On the cardiovascular system:

Fasting reduces bad cholesterol, regulates blood volume and normalises blood pressure. Animal research has shown that it makes the heart muscle more efficient and accelerates the growth of the heart's blood vessels. Systolic blood pressure is lower. There is also an improvement in coronary functions and cells.

On the kidneys and adrenals:

- Drainage of toxins throughout the body.
- Increased vitality.
- Increased production of hormones called catecholamines (adrenaline and noradrenaline).
- Increased production of corticosteroid hormones (cortisol, testosterone, progesterone, oestrogen).

On the immune system:

- Increased elimination of dysfunctional or defective immune system cells.
- Global restructuring of the immune system from three days.

Prolonged fasting can reinvent your immune system. When the body goes without food for a certain period of time, in order to conserve energy, it recycles diseased immune cells, giving you new strength to fight disease.

Rejuvenation

Research has shown that fasting slows down the ageing process in animals. The opinion is not yet clear-cut in humans, but many believe that fasting reduces free radicals, which are the main cause of ageing. Fasting is also thought to increase lifespan. When people fasted for five days, even on water, their secretion of growth hormone (GH) increased considerably. These results show that fasting can influence GH secretion and help the body adapt to famine.

Dr Rajeev Singh.

3. The nervous system and dry fasting

This dry fasting method is gaining in popularity, not least for its potential benefits for overall health and more specifically for the nervous system. In a world where neurological disorders are on the rise, due to a multitude of factors such as stress, poor diet, sedentary lifestyle, infections, electromagnetic pollution and excessive use of medication, the search for solutions to strengthen and restore our nervous system has become paramount.

Dry fasting could offer a promising way forward in this area, mainly because of its ability to induce deep detoxification of cells, including nerve cells. By abstaining from all food and water intake, the body is forced to draw on its internal reserves, leading to an accelerated elimination of accumulated toxins. This detoxification process could help to cleanse nerve cells, encouraging them to function optimally and helping to prevent degenerative diseases.

One of the most fascinating aspects of dry fasting is its ability to induce what are known as "renovative crises". These occur when the body, during the fasting phase, begins to actively expel toxins and repair damaged tissues. For these renovative crises to occur, dry fasting must be maintained for a sufficiently long period, which varies from person to person. These periods of crisis are often interpreted as a sign that the body is undergoing significant purification and regeneration, which could have a positive impact on the health of the nervous system.

In addition, sleep disorders, such as difficulty falling asleep or non-restorative sleep, can be the first signs of chronic neurological disorders. Dry fasting, by improving sleep quality and reducing stress, can help reverse these warning signs and contribute to the prevention of chronic nervous disorders. Indeed, quality sleep is essential to allow the nervous system to rest and regenerate.

However, it is crucial to note that dry fasting is a demanding practice that is not suitable for everyone. Before undertaking dry fasting, it is imperative to consult a health professional in order to assess its feasibility and safety for each individual. People with pre-existing medical conditions, pregnant or breast-feeding women should exercise particular caution.

Finally, although the potential benefits of dry fasting on the nervous system are promising, research in this area is still in its infancy. More in-depth studies are needed to validate these effects and understand the underlying mechanisms. Nevertheless, testimonials and individual experiences suggest that dry fasting could be an interesting avenue for those seeking to improve their neurological health and prevent neurodegenerative disorders. We have seen this in many patients suffering from multiple sclerosis, Alzheimer's, Parkinson's or epilepsy in the early stages of the disease.

Dry fasting therefore offers an interesting prospect for the health of the nervous system, with the promise of deep detoxification, cellular regeneration and an improvement in general well-being.

4. Effects on viral, bacterial and parasitic infections

There are some studies in the literature indicating that wet fasting has a slight positive effect on certain bacteria, but nothing has been studied in clinical practice.
https://www.medicalnewstoday.com/articles/mouse-study-suggests-fasting-may-help-contain-some-infections

Based on my experience during the pandemic, I have successfully helped more than 20 people who developed Covid. In fact, three to four days of dry fasting completely halts a viral infection.

The effects are also remarkable on sinusitis and infectious sore throats. It's important to understand that bacteria feed on sugar and water, and if these are no longer present, nothing can proliferate. This method is unique and would have a definite impact on the whole field of infectiology, but nobody is really interested in it. We've also helped more than 15 people with Lyme disease, with positive results. It takes three full nights of dry fasting to stop an infectious phenomenon.

CHAPTER 15

The emotional and energetic effects of dry fasting

1. Psychological discomfort during dry fasting

Fasting is supposed to improve mood through ketone bodies, which are antidepressants. Depressive phases can occur because dry fasting pushes you into a state of discomfort and malaise that exacerbates your nervous system and the influx of circulating toxins modifies your mood, sometimes in a negative way. Repressed feelings from the past may surface, as may repressed grief. This should be seen as an opportunity for renewal and for putting into words what you are feeling during dry fasting.

2. Feeling and introspection

It is essential to take note of how you feel and your emotional and mental state during this period. Dry fasting is not just a physical practice, but also a profound introspective experience. Take the time to note how you feel inside each day, and observe any changes in your self-perception and emotional state. If dreams and compulsive eating return, this is a sign of physical and mental detoxification.

Careful monitoring of these constants will give you a better understanding of how your body reacts to dry fasting. This will help you to make informed decisions about continuing or stopping fasting, depending on your state of health. It is crucial to remember that dry fasting should be practised with caution and, ideally, under competent supervision, especially if you are new to the practice or have pre-existing health problems.

3. The three phases of inner work during the seven-nine day dry fast

- **Phase 1: Initial elimination of waste and body reactions**

During this initial phase, the body begins to adjust to the lack of food and water intake and, above all, to detoxify significantly. This phase lasts a maximum of three to four days for dry fasting and seven days for water fasting. Water fasting can be compared to a post office counter where there is a large crowd but only one assistant available. In this analogy, the "customers" are the toxins and waste that the body begins to mobilise for elimination. But there's only one counter available and lots of customers piling up. The "window" represents the body's elimination pathways, principally the blood and lymph, which transport waste to the elimination organs such as the kidneys, lungs, intestines and liver. If these pathways are congested or inefficient, waste elimination will be slow, leading to a variety of symptoms such as headaches, aches and pains, high pulse rates and multiple aches and pains, which are often the sign of an accumulation of toxins on the body's surface.

For beginners to dry fasting, anxiety can arise because the body doesn't know how to react to the unknown situation of having no liquid or solid intake. It can be disturbing not knowing what will happen physically and mentally. All that lost nervous energy can hamper detoxification. This first phase is the most difficult because it also corresponds to the metabolic switch from external food to internal food and the transition to ketosis, which occurs three times faster than in water fasting.

In some cases, a sensation of cold may occur during this phase, but this will disappear from the fourth day onwards. In short, this phase removes surface toxins. If you have not prepared your food properly, or if you have eaten poor-quality industrial food just before the dry fast, you could be in a lot of trouble. Some people stop their dry fasting after three days because they feel too unwell. But this has nothing to do with dry fasting, which people always try to pass off as dangerous or inappropriate, when it's simply a case of too many toxins in circulation and emunctories that are too weak. Low vitality does not allow toxins to be expelled.

- **Phase 2: Intensification of elimination and associated symptoms**

In the second phase, from the third to the fifth day, which corresponds to the second week of water fasting, the body intensifies its efforts to purge itself of accumulated waste, which can lead to kidney pains, vomiting and other various symptoms affecting the liver and intestines. But the symptoms will be less severe than during the first phase. This generally occurs around the fourth day of dry fasting. We can imagine that the body's 'motorways' are now open, allowing a smoother flow of toxins to the organs of elimination. This is also the very beginning of organ renewal, as autophagy begins to peak and so does ketosis. Fat is being consumed and growths, cysts or lumps are gradually beginning to dissolve. Remember that noble tissues (liver, brain, heart) are never affected. The kidneys begin to purify by autophagy, facilitating the expulsion of crystals and kidney stones, while gallstones may soften and dissolve.

- **Phase 3: Functional restructuring and** harmonisation

From the fifth to the tenth day of dry fasting, this phase is crucial, equivalent to the third or fourth week of a water fast. It marks the time for functional restructuring, physiological and organic re-harmonisation, and above all, increased production of stem cells and growth hormones. These play a key role in the renewal of the body as a whole. The regeneration process initiated by dry fasting can continue for a period of one to three weeks after it has ended.

Dry fasting, especially when practised over an extended period of seven to ten days, passes through three essential phases which can theoretically simulate or accelerate certain detoxification processes and contribute to the healing of chronic pathologies. The unique and remarkable curative effect of dry fasting is often attributed to the second acidosis crisis. However, the majority of fasters rarely reach this critical phase.

This last stage also involves deep introspection and an assessment of one's own limits. Mental control becomes paramount. It is crucial to remain focused on one's own journey without allowing oneself to be influenced by the experiences of others in a group. Although this phase can be marked by silence, certain crises can occur as early as day 7, making day 6 particularly trying. It is often at this point that many fasters, especially on the first dry fast, feel extremely tired and decide to stop.

This phase can be seen as one of complete restructuring of the human being. The testimonies of those who have undertaken several long successive fasts confirm this: the signs of rejuvenation are visible, with darker hair and a face visibly younger than its initial state. This transformation attests to the power of dry fasting as a tool for body regeneration and overall revitalisation.

4. How does therapeutic dry fasting work on a person's energy?

Therapeutic dry fasting has a two-way effect on energy. On the one hand, it eliminates energy blockages, including negative aspects and illnesses. On the other, it encourages the accumulation of new, healthier energy. Many practitioners, such as mediums and tarot readers, observe the evacuation of substances such as grey smoke, energy links and various waste products during prolonged dry fasting. This is confirmed by modern technical devices that allow these energetic processes to be partially observed.

Even without adhering to these beliefs, it is common for people to lose the desire to consume alcohol, tobacco or even drugs after a long dry fast. This change occurs not for philosophical or spiritual reasons, but because the addiction fades and is replaced by a natural aversion, following the cleansing of the body. What's more, after a period of fasting, a transformation in eating habits is often observed, with a rejection of unhealthy foods such as junk food, or even meat. The taste buds seem to regenerate, making healthy foods more appetising and unhealthy ones more unpalatable.

Abstinence from food is also a powerful way of pacifying the mind, surpassing all other methods. This practice allows us to manage our thoughts about hunger differently, encouraging a more detached and less compulsive reaction to bodily signals. Fasting also increases energy reserves, a phenomenon that may seem paradoxical. Deprived of biological nourishment, the body intensifies its absorption of subtle energy from space and the environment, leading to a surplus of energy once normal eating is resumed.

Fasting also has a purifying effect on the chakras and energy channels, influencing various abilities and reducing the need for sleep. However, these benefits can be compromised if fasting is not accompanied by a healthy lifestyle, including a balanced diet, physical exercise and time spent outdoors in the sunshine.

The dry fasting process can be accompanied by an intensification of emotions, which can be surprising and unsettling, especially for beginners. It is crucial to work on your emotions during dry fasting, to share them and to bring them to the surface of your consciousness. This is what we have put in place in our retreats, in order to transform the negative into the positive and prevent fasting from turning into a form of self-torture. We recommend that you become aware of your emotions, analyse them and accept them, rather than fighting or repressing them. By doing so, we achieve a state of energetic and emotional purification, which is essential for maximising the benefits of therapeutic fasting.

5. Emotional-energetic purification during dry fasting.

By freeing ourselves from emotional toxins, we open the door to a deeper understanding of ourselves and explore new states of being. This helps us to dive more deeply into our inner world. Dry fasting, particularly when practised over a long period, offers a unique opportunity to reveal our predominant emotions and feelings. During this period, these emotions manifest themselves more clearly because, without the possibility of 'feeding' on external distractions, our ego can no longer conceal them. This process makes visible on our faces and in our behaviour what we usually try to hide.

Discovering the feelings we repress in our daily lives allows us to transform them, even after we have completed the dry fast. In this way, we can enrich our soul and body with positive energy and use it for the good of ourselves and others. Dry fasting is particularly beneficial for those who tend to compensate for their negative emotions with food. Emotions such as boredom, stress, resentment, anxiety and worry often lead to overeating. Dry fasting encourages us to reflect on the real reasons behind our desire to eat, distinguishing physical hunger from fears and emotions. This practice is therefore an excellent way of combating emotional overeating.

Emotional and energetic cleansing is crucial, especially for those who interact frequently with others. Emotional exhaustion syndrome, common among professionals such as educators, doctors, consultants, journalists, sales managers and social workers, results from the accumulation of negative energies exchanged during interactions. Long-term dry fasting can effectively eliminate these accumulated negative energies, both our own and those of others.

Finally, fasting promotes a transition towards "internal nutrition", offering profound peace to the nervous system. It allows deep, prolonged relaxation, contributing to a healthier, calmer mental state. In short, dry fasting is more than just a physical exercise; it is a profound practice of emotional healing and self-discovery.

6. Fasting and the emotions: a deep connection for healing

Dry fasting plays a crucial role in the relationship between our bodies and our emotions. This ancient practice, recognised for its benefits to physical health, also has a profound impact on our emotional well-being. By choosing to fast, we embark on an inner journey of discovery and healing.

Dry fasting creates a unique environment for the body and mind. One of the fascinating theories linked to dry fasting is that of the elimination of water with engrammed information. According to this theory, the water we consume on a daily basis can carry emotional imprints and memories, contributing to our overall emotional state. During a period of dry fasting, this 'informed' water would be eliminated, making way for the pure metabolic water produced by the body itself. This internal purification process can lead to a release of engrammed emotions, providing a form of deep emotional cleansing.

Fasting provides an opportunity to confront buried emotions and past traumas. By depriving the body of its usual routines, fasting triggers an introspective process, enabling individuals to confront their emotions and process them in a more conscious and healthy way. This confrontation often leads to a feeling of emotional release and a renewed sense of emotional balance.

7. Dry fasting: a tool for rebalancing emotions

As well as its effects on physical health, fasting serves as a tool for rebalancing the emotions. It teaches us to listen to our bodies and respond to our needs in a more harmonious way. This rebalancing leads to greater self-understanding and emotional stability.

In conclusion, dry fasting is a powerful practice that goes beyond physical purification. It offers a pathway to emotional healing and emotional balance, helping us to release engrained emotions and establish a deeper connection with our inner being.

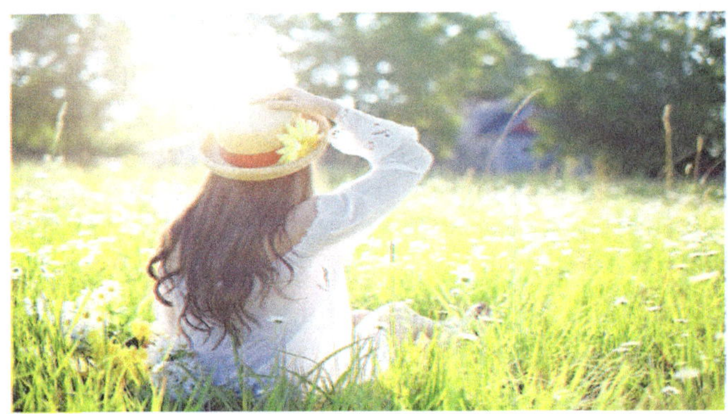

8. Finding a purpose in life helps happiness and healing

Finding a purpose in life is an essential quest that goes to the heart of human existence. This search for meaning goes far beyond the satisfaction of material needs or personal ambitions: it's about self-realisation and inner happiness. Having a clear purpose can act as a guide, directing choices, actions and priorities through the challenges and uncertainties of life. What's more, aligning oneself with deep, personal meaning can be a powerful key to healing and well-being. The link between purpose and happiness is strong. Happiness here is more than just fleeting joy or immediate pleasure; it is a deep and lasting contentment, fuelled by the conviction that we are living a meaningful and important life. Positive psychology research has shown that people with a clear sense of purpose tend to enjoy better mental health, are more resilient to stress and experience higher levels of life satisfaction.

The quest for purpose is highly personal and can take many forms. For some, it may involve contributing to society, whether through their profession, volunteering or artistic expression. For others, it may be the pursuit of knowledge, spiritual exploration, or the creation of deep and meaningful relationships. The important thing is to discover what resonates most intimately, what brings satisfaction and fulfilment.

Inner happiness plays a crucial role in physical and mental healing. The positive state of mind that comes from a sense of purpose can improve the immune system, speed recovery from illness and reduce the perception of pain. Mentally, it can help combat depression, anxiety and other emotional disorders. This is why more and more holistic health practices are incorporating the search for meaning and the development of inner happiness into their healing approaches.

To find your purpose, it's helpful to engage in introspection, engage in different activities to discover what sparks enthusiasm and motivation, get fully involved in the area of meaning you've identified, build meaningful relationships with others who share your values, and cultivate gratitude and mindfulness to stay anchored in the present. By pursuing what gives deep meaning to your life, you pave the way for a more fulfilled and harmonious existence, where inner happiness is both the path and the destination, creating a virtuous circle of well-being and healing.

9. Dry fasting as a gateway to spiritual healing, the awakening of consciousness and the evolution of the being

Dry fasting is proving to be an ancient practice of exceptional depth, offering far more than physiological benefits. This discipline emerges as a path of integral purification, conducive to spiritual healing and a powerful opening of consciousness that few words can explain.

At the heart of this practice, the lack of water pushes the fasting person to the very depths of their inner self. It is in this denial, this conscious deprivation, that hidden dimensions of our being are revealed. Deprived of the most basic elements of survival, the body enters a state of deep purification, releasing not only physical toxins, but also emotional and mental burdens accumulated over time and years, and even trans-generational burdens.

The mental clarity that emerges from this process goes beyond a simple cognitive improvement. The brain, relieved of the burden of digestion, opens up to levels of thought and reflection that are often unexplored and unknown. It's an amplified state of mind, an open window on the unknown, where understanding of oneself and the world takes on a new dimension.

Lack of water, by pushing the fasting person to the threshold of resilience, becomes an exceptional catalyst for opening up consciousness. Mystics throughout the ages have often experienced states of transcendence during periods of conscious deprivation. The doors of spiritual connection are then opened, revealing profound inner truths and giving rise to unforgettable mystical experiences.

Dry fasting, much more than a simple deprivation, thus becomes a powerful tool for the evolution of our Being. The individual, confronted with his or her own physical and mental limits, embarks on a journey of self-discovery. Repressed emotions and deep-seated thoughts all come to the surface, creating fertile ground for daring inner exploration.

In this exploration, abstinence becomes a means of transcending the ordinary dimensions of reality. Deprived of material restraints, the fasting person plunges into an altered state of consciousness where perceptions of time, space and self are altered in extraordinary ways. This inner transformation, often described as a spiritual rebirth, is the very foundation of the evolution of our Being.

By embracing this practice with calm, acceptance of what is happening with respect and kindness, individuals can not only experience physical regeneration, but also explore uncharted inner territory. Dry fasting thus becomes a pathway to profound self-evolution and an awakening of consciousness that transcends the limitations of everyday life.

Beyond these initial benefits, this age-old discipline is an integral experience of spiritual healing, awakening of consciousness and evolution of Being. However, the real essence of the transformation is revealed when you emerge from the dry fast, where it's important to maintain an attitude of gratitude and wonder.

Once the fast is over, the body enters a phase of profound renewal. The organs revitalised by fasting function at full capacity, eliminating accumulated residues and stimulating cell regeneration. This cellular rebirth extends to all the organs, strengthening the immune system and laying the foundations for optimal health.

Repressed emotions, released during the fast, can be confronted and processed consciously, leading to greater emotional stability and a deeper understanding of the self. At the heart of this experience lies personal rebirth. Dry fasting, combined with post-fasting cleansing, offers the opportunity to rid oneself of old habits, limiting thought patterns and stagnant energies. It's a chance to deliberately redefine our being, to shape a better version of ourselves.

Cure Recipes: Food Reintroduction.

10. Food Reintroduction after Dry Fasting - Key to Therapeutic Effectiveness

The phase of food resumption after dry fasting is without doubt the most crucial stage in guaranteeing the success and therapeutic effectiveness of fasting. Contrary to what many people might think, the fasting period itself represents only a fraction of the whole process. In fact, over 80% of the benefits depend on how you gradually reintroduce food into your diet. This chapter focuses on the importance of this phase, explaining the basic principles and providing concrete examples to guide you.

Why is Food Recovery so Essential?

During a dry fast, your body goes through an in-depth cleansing, intense cellular detoxification and metabolic regeneration. When you come out of fasting, your digestive system is in a particularly sensitive and vulnerable state. Reintroducing food abruptly or inappropriately could not only cancel out the benefits obtained, but also cause digestive problems, metabolic imbalances and even inflammation.

Reintroducing food is therefore an opportunity to stabilise and reinforce the therapeutic gains achieved during fasting. It should be gentle, gradual and respectful of the work done by your body. The choice of food, the way it is prepared and eaten, and the timing of its introduction are all determining factors.

During my travels in Russia, I witnessed many monumental errors in the resumption of eating after a group dry fast. I often observed food orgies where foods were consumed excessively and without any consideration for their compatibility. Within the first two or three days of resumption, some people were already complaining of digestive problems, which is extremely problematic. This compromises not only all the effort invested during the fast, but also the expected benefits. A haphazard resumption of eating can really cancel out the positive effects of fasting and cause discomfort that could have been avoided with a more controlled approach to the food given.

The Key Principles of Eating After a Dry Fast

1. **Avoiding Carbohydrates and Sugary Products for the First 7 Days:** It is crucial to avoid carbohydrates, sweet products

and any food or drink with a sweet taste, even if they are natural, for the first 7 days. As the body is in an advanced state of detoxification, the premature introduction of carbohydrates could trigger intestinal fermentation and imbalances in the flora.

2. **Respect the Food Progression:** The resumption of eating follows a precise structure. Start with light liquids such as broths or diluted soups, before moving on to purées or steamed vegetables, followed by light proteins and healthy fats. Solid foods should be introduced gently, observing the body's reactions at each stage.

3. **Personalising the recovery according to your profile:** Although the first stages are broadly similar for everyone, the rest of the recovery must be personalised according to your bioresonance check-up carried out before the cure, your constitution, your metabolism, your digestion and the way your fasting went. Your professional activity, your specific nutritional needs and your pace of life also influence the food choices to be made.

4. **Listen to your body and observe how you feel:** During this phase, it's essential to listen to your body. Introduce new foods gradually and in small quantities, taking care to chew well and to feel the effects of each meal on your digestion. This will help you to detect any intolerances or sensitivities.

Conference on Eating Again: A Personalised Guide

In the conference I offer at the end of the retreat, all these concepts are discussed in detail. Together we analyse the best nutritional strategies for your profile and your health goals. You'll leave with a clear roadmap and tailored advice for the period following your dry fast. This will make it easier to determine what diet is best for you during the two months of transition that follow.

1. **Delicate Courgette or Radish Soup (Day 1 or 2)**
   This simple, gentle soup is ideal for reintroducing food. Boil courgettes or radishes in filtered water, without adding salt. Once the vegetables are cooked, blend until the texture is neither too liquid nor too thick. You can also use fennel, chicory or celery, but make sure you only blend one vegetable at a time for better digestion. When tasting, take the time to chew well and swirl each spoonful in your mouth before swallowing.

2. **Savoury Vegetable Chunky Soup (From Day 2)**
   From the second day back on the diet, opt for a soup with a few chunks of vegetables. Combine 2 to 3 of the following vegetables: fennel, endives, celery, green beans, courgettes, bamboo shoots, hearts of palm, bean sprouts, lettuce, olives, pumpkin, red pepper, chard, spinach, squash, rutabaga or turnip. The soup is made with just water and vegetables, without salt or oil. Serve this comforting soup in a pretty bowl for a light, nourishing meal.

3. **Steamed or Boiled Vegetables (Quick Cook - 10 minutes)**
   From the second day onwards, serve vegetables steamed or boiled in water for a maximum of 10 minutes. Arrange them attractively on a serving dish, taking into account the number of guests. Recommended vegetables include: fennel, endives, celery, green beans, courgettes, bamboo shoots, hearts of palm, bean sprouts, lettuce, olives, pumpkin, red pepper, chard, spinach, squash, rutabaga, turnip. Gentle cooking preserves the natural flavour and texture of the vegetables.

4. **Fish and Vegetable Soup (Day 3 and beyond)**
   Prepare a light soup with boneless fish and 2 to 3 vegetables of your choice from the list above. Gently

simmer the fish with the vegetables to extract all the flavours. This nutritious soup is perfect for gentle digestion while providing quality protein. Choice of small fish.

5. **Lightly Whitened Konjac (Day 2 or 3)**
   From the second or third day, introduce small quantities of konjac. Cook the konjac for 2 minutes in boiling water, then serve it as a side dish. From the fifth day onwards, you can add a light sauce prepared with organic herbs, coconut cream and water.

6. **Quail eggs (Days 2 to 5)**
   Start with 1 raw or cooked quail egg on the second day. Gradually increase the quantity to 3 eggs a day from the third day onwards. From the fifth day, depending on your digestion, you can introduce conventional eggs in small quantities. Make sure you chew each mouthful well for better assimilation. The scissors are supplied with the treatment.

7. **Remineralisation and Kidney Drainage Nettle Herbal Tea (1 to 3 days)**
   Infuse nettle in boiling water for 10 minutes, then strain. Consume this hot tea for three days following the end of dry fasting to provide essential minerals.

8. **Oven Roasted Vegetables (From Day 3)**
   Choose from a variety of vegetables to roast: romaine or iceberg lettuce, baby spinach, cucumber (without skin or seeds), courgettes, green beans, aubergine (without skin), peppers, celery, watercress, endives, Chinese cabbage (bok choy), radishes. Baking enhances the natural flavours of the vegetables while preserving their delicate texture.

Recommended supplements :

1. **Régulat pro bio (natural probiotic)**: 1/2 teaspoon in 200 ml of water in the morning on an empty stomach for 2 days. For people with sensitive digestion, 10 drops are enough.
2. **Homemade Spirulina**: Add to your soup or mix 1 teaspoon in a glass of water from the second day. If all goes well, gradually increase to 2 teaspoons a day after a week.
3. **Pianto**: From 4-5 days after starting to drink again, take 1 teaspoon a day to support intestinal transit if necessary. It is normal not to have any bowel movements for the first few days following a dry fast.
4. **Fir resin**: Recommended to remineralise and alkalinise the body after fasting. Start with small doses and gradually increase.

Very important: No carbohydrates, sweet products, drinks or solid foods, or sweet-tasting fruit for the first 7 days following the end of the dry fast.

Conclusion: Optimal Eating Recovery for Lasting Health

The dietary resumption phase is a delicate but extremely beneficial period when properly managed. This is where the power of dry fasting lies. By following these principles and adapting the strategy to your specific needs, you will optimise the therapeutic effectiveness of dry fasting while supporting your body in a smooth transition to a balanced diet.

CHAPTER 16

The return to love, a path to healing

by Marie Christine Millet, life practitioner of therapeutic dry fasting with Michel Deladoey

In this chapter, we're going to look at some of the Hermetic* principles[1] which are designed to help us better understand the mechanism of illness. In addition to having an effect on our physical body through dysfunctions that bring out pain and aches, we are also going to bring together aches and pains through words, by means of an understanding and global awareness of being. The being is "who I am" in the physical body (matter), the heart-soul (through emotions), the state of mind (mental programmes) and the spirit-divine (access to universal consciousness).

We are touching on a vast subject which, in all humility, would deserve thousands of lifetimes to extract its essence. An overview is transmitted to me through an innate knowledge. It obviously remains a truth of its own, based on observation of a large number of people in the context of coaching, in the professional and personal spheres, as well as during my many

---

[1] * *The Hermetic Laws are a set of philosophical and esoteric principles attributed to the Hermetic tradition, which has its roots in the teachings attributed to Hermes Trismegistus, a mythical figure of antiquity. These laws are often presented in texts such as the «Kybalion», published in the early 20th century. Hermes Trismegistus is often associated with wisdom, esoteric knowledge and spiritual healing. His teachings, transmitted through texts such as the Corpus Hermeticum, deal with concepts related to health and well-being.*

travels. I hope you will discover an authentic and neutral vision of the whole being and its innate capacity for self-healing.

We are going to detect what evil has to tell us (illness = evil said), by learning to become explorers of our "being". In fact, it's by really delving into our depths and our pain that we're going to undertake a formidable initiation into what we originally are.

My aim is to help you gain a more spiritual understanding of what illness can teach us, using the universal laws of Hermetic philosophy as a parallel.

One of the Hermetic principles refers to the law of correspondence, i.e. *"whatever is above is like whatever is below, and whatever is below is like whatever is above"*. Obviously, we're talking about the matter that makes up our physical body, but we're also talking about the spirit, which is our energetic body. This means that when we heal our physical body, we also heal our energy body and vice versa. When this principle is evoked in the context of illness, it brings us back to an understanding of the similarity between the visible and the invisible on two planes of consciousness that are different in perception, yet unified when we understand the mechanics. In particular, what we see through our senses (projection towards the outside world) and what happens inside us (inner observation), which I'm going to call feelings or listening to oneself.

The law of correspondence, which is not always easy to understand, I grant you, exists to enable us to confirm whether what we perceive through our senses corresponds to what we feel through the prism of our intuition. This validation leads us to a profound state of fullness, lightness and joy, which is nothing other than a deep understanding and unity in 'who I am'. Conversely, when there is a 'false' interpretation between what I perceive and what I feel, it leads to vibratory dissonance, a separating state and a disproportionate and heightened emotional reaction. Hence the importance of not stifling our emotions but observing them, without judgement, to try to understand what has generated a wound, a fault, a pain inside us that is responsible for creating the emotion. Because the real cause of any illness is none other than a misinterpretation of a situation which, by dint of repetition, leads us to accumulate a high level of stress. This, then, is the cause of all physical and energetic dysfunction, which has given rise to the majority of our ailments, which are simply their effect.

And this is where our true initiation begins, to discover our being, in other words "who I am", through a heroic journey to unify our two parts and free ourselves from this feeling of separation or rather isolation between who I am inside and the way I perceive the outside world. At that point, total healing takes place.

Why do I think it's important to stress this point? Because I think it's obvious that to achieve lasting healing, we need to look after our bodies and minds by observing our emotions. And it's not by repressing them or trying to control them through superficial methods that we'll be able to free ourselves from our ills.

1. The first door to healing: the intelligence of the soul's heart, its emotions

Within us there is a source of wisdom, a remarkable intelligence that enables us to solve all our problems or ailments if we know how to listen to it. Throughout history, this intelligence has been revealed by the Latin word "motio" or "emotio", which, according to Cicero or Seneca, meant the passions of the soul. They are associated with notions of virtue and reason. It is a moral force that pushes our being towards good (the opposite polarity to evil) by applying itself to following moral laws.

As we said earlier, illness is a disharmony, an inner imbalance. "Mal a dit" means that within us is evil, pain, which it will be fundamental to reverse through the law of polarity (second hermetic principle) by turning towards the good to regain our well-being. It's a principle of balance that we can either deny or integrate.

So our emotions are a message from the heart that generates behaviour? It is also the link between our inner world and the representation we make of it on the outside. If we are too focused on the outside world, physical illness manifests itself, while on the other hand, too much introspection can plunge us into mental illness. We are going to return to harmony by cultivating a more positive life that is more attuned to ourselves.

Emotions are nothing more than a revelation of our world as a whole and the direction of our energy. They are our own intelligence which, like a compass, enables us to find our inner balance. Emotions can be classified into several categories, including joy, sadness, fear, anger, disgust and surprise, although the exact list may vary according to psychological theories and researchers.

We will not go into the details and complexity of the link between emotion and illness. Although emotions can be adaptive and normal responses to certain situations (imminent danger, for example), research has shown that they can also act as **causes** of illness, such as:

- Chronic stress (weakens the immune system, increases inflammation in the body and contributes to the development of diseases such as cardiovascular disease, diabetes and gastrointestinal disorders),
- Negative and destructive behaviours (overeating, excessive alcohol consumption, smoking or lack of exercise),
- Stifling your emotions (increased risk of cardiovascular disease, gastrointestinal problems and mental disorders).

But also as **effects** that will exacerbate the disease:

- the psychological impact of a chronic or fatal illness,
- chronic pain, which aggravates its perception and can create a vicious circle,
- the physiological effects of chronic illnesses that affect the immune system, the nervous system and other bodily functions.

So here we come to a third hermetic principle, the law of causality. "*Every effect has a cause and every cause has an effect*". It is because, whether unconsciously or consciously, we experience a feeling of unease and judge it as bad, that illness sets in. It is our emotions that are the indicators, following a reaction or behaviour in relation to an event. We might therefore think that emotion is the effect at the origin of behaviour and thought the cause.

For example, if I feel bad about my life because I have a job that I don't like, but I convince myself that my situation is acceptable (in short, I'm lying to myself) because deep down I'm afraid of changing, of finding myself in a disastrous financial situation and on top of that I don't know what job I might like, I can trigger a form of chronic depression. The cause could be thinking that I have no solution to events and that my only choice is to stay in this situation. The effect would be a state of depression that could lead me to lower my immune system to the point of triggering chronic illnesses, for example, because I'm afraid to leave my comfort zone and I don't know how to get out of it. This will attract other complicated situations into my life, as if an influx of problems were materialising that generate ever more fear and ultimately sadness. It's as if my original thinking was wrong because it's leading me towards more and more disasters in my life and more and more strong emotions. But who actually created this? If not myself, by accepting a job that I don't like or by persevering in this job without trying to find another path...

What if an internal process was trying to set in motion, simply to warn me? A strong feeling that is trying to manifest itself in my life by setting off an intentional fire inside me. What if I hadn't taken the right path? In any case, not the one that I want, deep down inside. It's as if part of me knows what's good for me but I'm not listening.

So we're going to explore the notion of cause and effect in more depth by talking about the HeartMath Institute (an American institute based in California and set up in 1991). This institute has conducted research into the link between the heart, the brain, emotions and stress. The Heart Math Institute studied the two-way communication between the heart and the brain. They discovered that the heart sends electromagnetic signals to the brain that can influence cognitive, emotional and behavioural processes.

Using a panel of a large number of people, they carried out this study by noticing that the participants' heart rate changed a few seconds before they saw an image projected onto a video screen. This image was intended to trigger a cognitive, emotional and behavioural response. The surprise was to realise that the heart rate adopted exactly the heartbeat appropriate to the image presented on the video screen even before the participant was informed of it.

This could mean that the information was already there... but that the emotional reaction is activated a few seconds before the image is presented to us and interpreted by our brain. The cause would therefore be an invisible intelligence called the intelligence of the heart-soul. This intelligence already knows in advance what is going to happen. In fact, how many times have we gone to events where we knew perfectly well that something inside us was telling us not to go and a disaster occurred or the evening was a fiasco? This intelligence of the heart that some people call "intuition" is nothing more than a feeling that goes beyond our mental capacity to understand. Our brain interprets the information only at a later stage.

Emotion would therefore only be an effect. The cause would come from a form of intelligence other than our brain, a remarkable source of intelligence: the soul.

So how do some people manage to live serenely and remain in good health, while others are constantly reacting and are so energetically abused that they end up in a vicious circle of illness?

These people have succeeded in becoming masters of themselves by learning to listen to themselves, to understand this intelligence of the heart and to let it work through them. This is what we call unconditional love or "flow". It's a self-love that soothes the emotions and shows us the way to inner fulfilment, or in other words: being in tune with who I am and what I'm experiencing.

Why is it important to understand this before starting a dry fast? Because it will be necessary to prepare before starting such a process. Dry fasting is in fact the oldest method there is, the most direct route to healing that we call the dry way, the method for people who really want to explore the depths of their being and return to perfect health of body and mind.

This method will bring out all our mental programmes, our emotional reactions and act directly on our bodily pains. It will purify the body in all its dimensions if we agree to observe ourselves and allow ourselves to be guided. Doing a dry fast without going inside ourselves, into our feelings, without understanding them, will not allow any illness to disappear for good. Let's be honest, the illness will undeniably return after a few months. You will have had a few weeks or months of reprieve, enough to make your mouth water. Then it will be necessary to persevere until you fully understand "who I am".

To finish this part before the practice, let's not forget the most important thing: when our cells divided during our creation in the foetus, the first organ they created was the heart. So this part of us is much more important than anything we can imagine.

In the meantime, to understand the mechanism of the disease, it will be necessary to soothe our mental and emotional ailments in order to begin our journey. And this involves a whole range of exercises that can considerably improve your life.

1.1 Relaxation exercises

- **First exercise – Reduce emotional stress quickly – The basis for exploring your world.**

I defy anyone in the middle of a storm to take care of him. We can't! We're in survival mode. So we need to calm down, observe ourselves and learn to listen to ourselves, and here's the first exercise for calming our emotions when we're reacting. It's called cardiac coherence. This method is child's play, but all you need to do is learn the basics and make it part of your daily routine. You can download an application on your smartphone such as:

Petit bambou, Respirelax+, Respire®, Deep Belief, Mind, Cardiac Coherence, etc...

The ideal posture for successful cardiac coherence is to put yourself in a confident posture, i.e. shoulders slightly back, heart forward, back straight and head slightly down. Sit on the edge of a chair or on a cushion, letting your lower back take its place naturally. The aim is to have the sensation of being held by a thread above your head. The posture should not be painful; on the contrary, there should be a feeling of lightness and balance. The important thing is that you can relax completely in this position.

Breathing in is always from the bottom up, starting from the belly. The belly is inflated, then the diaphragm, and finally the ribcage up to the shoulder blades. You then have two options: either breathe out from the bottom, or from the top. By breathing out from the bottom upwards, you will raise the energy in your body. For people who are tired, this has the advantage of energising an exhausted body. But for those who prefer to calm down, it's better to breathe out from the top downwards.

The application will help you focus your attention on an element that appears on your smartphone. Either a bubble that rises and falls, or one that inflates and deflates to accompany your breathing and calm your agitated thoughts.

You'll need to practise this exercise at least twice a day, for five minutes in the first month, then ten minutes in the second and 15 minutes thereafter. It's a wonderful tool that will calm your emotions and your mind, and help you prepare for the rest of the exercises.

- **Second exercise – Connecting to the heart of the self through mindfulness meditation accompanied by binaural sounds**

Meditation, whether sitting or walking slowly, is a practice that consists of being fully aware of the present moment, paying open, non-judgemental attention to our bodily sensations, thoughts, emotions and environment.

The sitting meditation posture is generally simple and comfortable, encouraging conscious attention without distraction. Here are the key elements of the posture:

1. **Sitting:** most practitioners choose to sit on a meditation cushion or a comfortable chair. The key is to maintain an upright, balanced posture, without being stiff or tense.
2. **Straight back:** the back is kept straight, but not stiff. This encourages alertness and presence, while allowing you to breathe freely and naturally.
3. **Head tilted slightly downwards:** the head is generally tilted slightly downwards, with the chin slightly tucked in to align the spine.
4. **Eyes closed or half-closed:** the eyes can be closed to concentrate more on inner sensations, or half-closed to maintain a certain connection with the environment.
5. **Hands:** the hands are placed comfortably on the knees or in the lap, with the palms facing downwards or upwards, according to the practitioner's preference.
6. **Relaxation:** it is important to relax as much as possible, releasing any tension in the body, particularly in the shoulders, face and jaw. The use of stretching movements and a bodyscan* will help you to practise over time.
7. **Stability:** The posture is stable and anchored, with the feet placed flat and firmly on the floor if you are sitting in a chair.

What should I choose between meditating on a meditation cushion or a chair? Many practitioners think that meditating requires sitting on a cushion. What they don't tell you is that this posture was adopted by the Tibetans because at the time they didn't have chairs. There are very few forests in Tibet, and consequently very little wood to make them. As a result, Tibetans are used to sitting on cushions from an early age. In Europe, on the other hand, we are used to sitting on a chair. It will therefore be more natural and less painful for our joints. But you won't be a bad practitioner, rest assured. Initially, meditation requires a great deal of kindness towards yourself and your body.

Sitting meditation allows you to consciously observe your own being. Observe our thoughts without becoming attached to them by returning to our natural breathing. Listen to ourselves and our environment in a state of non-attachment, while at the same time being fully present. Feeling inner movements and tensions to consciously restore calm while returning to our breathing.

Walking meditation is a very slow form of meditation that requires full attention to maintain balance while relaxing the muscles of the body. The body is relaxed and the bare feet (preferably) are stable and anchored with each step. This mindful walking invites you to return to your senses and your breathing, while remaining open to your surroundings. For people who are very active, walking meditation can be very challenging, because slowness is a source of frustration when we're in the hustle and bustle of life. The aim is not to be distracted by our environment, but to accept the movements of life without paying attention to them.

The practice of meditation is a necessary activity to immerse ourselves fully in the present moment and return to the essence of our being. It helps to reduce physical, emotional and mental stress, while improving concentration and mental clarity. It can be practised every day for 15 to 30 minutes. Practising cardiac coherence can be the first step in calming stress before moving on to meditation.

Here is a study carried out by Eileen Luders and colleagues in 2012. They examined differences in brain volume between experienced meditators and non-meditators. The results showed significant differences in several brain regions, including an increase in grey matter volume in areas associated with attention, emotional regulation and body perception.

Why incorporate binaural sounds into your practice?

Binaural sounds are a form of auditory stimuli that involve the use of two tones of slightly different frequency, presented simultaneously to each ear. When these two tones are perceived by the brain, they create an auditory illusion of a beat, known as a binaural beat, which is perceived as a third sound. This difference in frequency creates interference between the sound waves in the brain, leading to changes in the brain waves themselves.

For example, if a 200 Hz tone is presented to one ear and a 210 Hz tone is presented to the other ear, the brain will perceive a 10 Hz beat. This binaural beat is associated with specific brain frequencies, which can influence states of consciousness, levels of alertness and other mental processes.

Binaural sounds are often used for relaxation, meditation, improving concentration, promoting sleep and other practices designed to influence brain activity. They are broadcast through stereo headphones so that each ear receives a different tone, allowing the brain to perceive the binaural beat.

Here are some examples of commonly used binaural sounds:

Relaxation frequencies: binaural frequencies such as 5 Hz (**delta**), 10 Hz (**theta**) or 15 Hz (**alpha**) are often used to induce a state of deep relaxation, meditation or sleep.

Improved concentration: higher binaural frequencies, such as 10 Hz to 20 Hz (**alpha and low beta**), are often used to increase concentration, alertness and mental clarity.

Sounds for sleep: lower binaural frequencies, such as 1 Hz to 4 Hz (**delta**), are often used to promote deep, recuperative sleep.

Cognitive stimulation: binaural frequencies in the range 15 Hz to 30 Hz (**beta**) can be used to stimulate brain activity and promote mental alertness, creativity and problem-solving.

Emotional balance: some binaural sound recordings are designed to balance emotions, promote emotional well-being and reduce stress.

It is important to note that the effects of binaural sounds can vary from person to person, and that some people may be more sensitive or receptive to these stimuli than others.

A study published in the *Journal of Alternative and Complementary Medicine* in 2007 found that listening to binaural sounds for 60 days reduced levels of cortisol (a stress hormone) in participants, suggesting a beneficial effect on stress and anxiety.

Combining the practice of mindfulness with brainwave stimulation helps reduce thoughts and stress, and improves concentration and mental clarity, with very powerful results in just 60 days, if you make it part of your daily routine.

- **Third exercise – Practising "Smile gratitude" on a daily basis**

Who doesn't know the word "THANK YOU"? It's probably the third word we learn after Mum and Dad. Gratitude also has the ability to transform our body chemistry. When we give thanks for things, for others, for ourselves, for events as they are, a real transmutation takes place in our bodies. We no longer see the world in terms of combat, but in terms of learning. Our posture changes; it's as if our attention, which was mental, suddenly descends into the heart. Then the intelligence of the heart comes into play.

And smiling is the best way to transform our facial physiology. The smile is perceived by our brain. When we smile, it's impossible to think negatively. And do you know why? Because our brain associates negative thoughts with bodily stress. So it creates a bug. At first it may be forced. Then it will become a habit until joy and calm return to your life.

So, wake up every morning with a smile on your face and thank yourself for being alive. If you're not satisfied with your life, give thanks as if your ideal life were manifesting itself in your life right now.

2. The path of the mind – The labyrinth: the importance of freeing the mind and undoing beliefs

The very first Hermetic principle tells us that *"All is spirit; the Universe is Mental"*. This is the principle of mentalism. It is fundamental to understand that everything that is outwardly apparent (to our material senses) is mental. Our world or the universe is therefore simply a mental creation of the "All". And it is in this universal and infinite mind that we live, act and are ourselves.

To simplify our understanding of the mind, we will try to find a very simplified form of correspondence with a computer. When we are in front of our screen, it projects images, stories and numbers. Depending on the software we have, which I will call beliefs or thoughts, we will be able to use our computer and achieve things. We will interpret the information we receive according to the data we have. What's interesting is that a simple computer is a very good mirror for understanding our inner mechanisms.

In this machine, software will be installed according to our culture, our family, our friends, our social level and many other factors. Some programmes are useful, but others will quickly become obsolete. Our brain also has a memory capacity to store all the information and make this mini world that appears on our inner screen work. This is our mind. Except that the world is changing so fast that a new factor has destabilised this tool. The creation of the web and its openness to the world has given rise to attacks, also known as viruses, which will weaken or even destroy our system. Computers have evolved and adapted to meet changing needs. Regular updates keep them working properly. By connecting to the web, we can access all the information of the past and present by accessing a network (matrix) that contains all the world's memory (for example, Google, but in spiritual language we speak of akashic memory).

The correspondence between our computer and the mechanics of our brain is quite striking. Except that our computer doesn't have the option of rejuvenating the parts, the memory is limited as soon as we start integrating too much information, the engine slows down from using too much software (programs) and we are increasingly obliged to add protection, firewalls, back-ups...

So what controls our computer? It's the motherboard, or rather our soul. It connects all the components, centralises the data and coding, and provides the power and resources our computer needs. In our body, and more particularly in our brain, it's our pineal gland that is the 'seat' of the soul. According to René Descartes, it is our mental control centre.

In short, by correspondence, the mind is all the programs, coding and storage contained in our brain. And what controls our mind is the throne of the soul, i.e. our pineal gland or pituitary gland.

Why is it important to understand this? Because if you feel blocked in your life, if you feel guilty, if you can't heal or whatever, it's because your programs, codes and memories don't allow your soul to feel free to be the most beautiful version of itself. So why do we have to judge ourselves so much, make ourselves suffer, fight so much in our daily lives?

Our mind has great power when we know how to use it properly, especially when we cleanse our pineal gland. To decalcify it, nothing is better than a diet free of sugar, caffeine, alcohol and tobacco. But chlorine, fluoride and bromide, as well as all the heavy metals contained in tap water, hygiene products and food, are also elements that block its proper functioning. Dr Joe Dispenza has carried out numerous studies on this gland, enabling many people to be completely cured by stimulating it through meditation and breathing practices.

We have seen that dry fasting is an extraordinary method for cell regeneration, but also for cleansing the control system of our mind, the seat of our soul. Meditation is also an incredible method for strengthening our brain power by activating neurogenesis. This is why we apply these two methods during our therapeutic dry fasting courses. Everyone unanimously talks about the incredible mental clarity we experience during a dry fasting process. Eating again is therefore fundamental to establishing healthy habits to maintain our mental faculties and keep our pituitary gland functioning properly.

So we have seen that our computer evolves like our mind as the world around us evolves. Our being adapts through this intelligence of life, a bit like an Artificial Intelligence in a computer that learns from its experiences while connecting to this collective memory. Except that AI doesn't have what's essential: a soul endowed with unlimited intelligence.

As a reminder, the mind is a bit like a seed and the life it contains, the soul. No creation is possible without the other. This seed already contains all the information about our DNA, our genes and our cells. This foetus will simply evolve and adapt according to our habits, our childhood and the programs we set up on our computer. We are born without any programs, blank. And it's the life we lead that will create the programs, beliefs, thoughts, history and identity that make us up.

The computer, the machine, is only the reflection of what we experience in a certain way in our mind, hence the importance of being aware that everything evolves in this world and that we cannot refuse change. To reject change is to lock ourselves in a cage or become obsolete. The only way to feel free is to open up our being and welcome what is. Our world is currently undergoing a magnificent transformation. Will we be able to see it as an act of love, or will we allow ourselves to be carried away by the fears that most often govern our lives?

All we have to do at this moment is simply say STOP to our fears! What if I learned to trust this world, or should I say "my" world, because I am the creator of my own world? Wouldn't that finally be the way to trust yourself to take the plunge into life? Relax, breathe deeply, imagine that in the centre of my chest my heart chakra is opening up so that I can now transform my limiting beliefs by accepting to take back the throne of my existence. Love is the key. The pineal gland, the power to transform your life.

Most of us are in survival mode without even realising it. Basically, we don't want our world to change. We cling to everything we know, our past, the objects and people around us. Letting go means accepting the transformation that is taking place. And the only way to create the future is not to reproduce the past... What do you think?

Regular meditation, a detox diet or fasting are all habits that can be cultivated to cleanse the pineal gland and bring more clarity into your life. Not to mention the many other benefits.

I don't want to shock you, but the reality is that our body is a very impressive biomechanical system that works like a computer. What distinguishes us from a machine is when our soul and our mind function in unity, because when they do, a much bigger door opens in us, the door of the Spirit, which has unfailing strength of will. But if we live in constant duality, then we can be influenced and manipulated like robots. Illness then becomes inevitable, because duality is the cause of all our ills. If you don't know which foot to dance on and someone tells you that the right foot will enable you to move forward more quickly, you're going to listen to them. Influence consists of putting doubt between your mind and the aspirations of your soul to the point where you only listen to others.

The mind also has the ability to quickly lose itself in a never-ending stream of thoughts. Depending on the kind of life we lead, our thoughts can be pleasant at best and unpleasant at worst. In fact, when they are pleasant, we can observe that our life becomes easier. We don't need to fight, the right people arrive at the right time, as if magic were happening in the invisible world to give us the opportunity to achieve everything we want. It's the soul that acts. On the other hand, our unpleasant thoughts will lead us into dead ends, walls and obstacles that will exhaust us. However, the moment when we feel at our best is when our brain loses track of time and we forget that we're thinking. For example, during an evening out with friends, when our mind is wandering. An emptiness that connects us to another, quieter part of ourselves, namely Spirit.

To conclude, what is the point of taking care of the seat of your soul and reuniting soul and mind? To no longer be under the control of external elements and to extricate ourselves from the labyrinth by rising above it. So let's regain control of our lives by letting our soul regain its sovereignty. It knows the path to unity. So we're going to practise a few exercises and routines to quickly calm our minds.

2.1 *Practical exercises*

- **Exercise 1: Clear your mental space by decluttering your life**

Everything that is inside me is also projected into the world in which I live. That's why it's important to free up your living space in the same way as you free up your mental space. Sort, give away, share, repair, get rid of broken objects and things you no longer wear. Clear your house. Clean your house, your garage, your car. Get out in the garden, get your hands in the soil or buy plants and look after them. Handicrafts can also calm the mind. Use your hands and give yourself time.

Everything you own is a reflection of what's inside you. Make room for the new. Create your own paradise. Home staging and vegetable gardening are excellent activities for those who don't have a lot of money! Use incense, burn sage and light candles to turn your home into a sanctuary, a temple of fulfilment where life is good. However, let the air into this space, ventilate it and open it up to the world. When we welcome the world as it is, it's important to have a pleasant place to recharge our batteries, not a cabin far from everything and cut off from the world. As the other is only a part of ourselves, rejecting them would only be a way of running away from ourselves.

If you tend to manage everything in your home, at work and elsewhere, why do you want to memorise everything in your brain? Write it down, make a to-do list. Jot it down, write it down, get unnecessary thoughts out of your brain. What's the point of keeping track of things, buying nappies, washing powder and milk, apart from cluttering up your brain? Writing it down in your diary or on paper frees up your mind considerably. Turn off the software on your computer, otherwise your brain will start to idle and roam. Then move your thoughts to the next sieve. Is this thought urgent? Is it important? If it's neither important nor urgent, what do you decide to do? Obligations or do you choose to simplify your life? It's all about choice. Take control of your life.

- **Second exercise: cultivate a philosophy of life that frees your mind, based on the four Toltec Agreements.**

Here are four phrases to nurture on a daily basis that can transform your life. These agreements are rules of life from the Toltec culture. You can always read the book written by Don Miguel Ruiz on the four Toltec agreements. We also apply these agreements in our dry fasting courses with Michel, because they really help to create a safe living space for each and every one of us.

1 - Your word must be impeccable

This is the most important and the most difficult to honour. Your words have both creative and destructive power. Did you know that the second organ created in the foetus after the heart is the tongue? Don't speak ill of others, because if you do, you're speaking ill of yourself. In the Old Testament, it is said that the "Word" or "Logo" is the creator. This means exactly the same thing. If you're used to grumbling, listen to yourself rather than just complaining, and change what you don't like about your life. Life is perpetual change, impermanence. Why not change your life if it doesn't suit you? No one can do it for you.

2 - Whatever happens, don't take it personally
You're not responsible for what other people say or do, even if it's directed at you. Everyone has their own personal truth and it's OK to disagree. However, we are responsible if we feel hurt by what others say, because it builds on a pain that is already there. Otherwise, we would not be affected. But why does the hurt exist? Because we reject what we feel instead of accepting the learning that is passed on to us. The wound allows the light to penetrate our spirit. Let life touch us, let us be vulnerable so that we can grow. When a muscle grows, it tears. When a tree grows, its bark stretches and tears. This is not pain, but wisdom and maturity.

3 - Don't make assumptions
Sometimes we are too quick to interpret situations and things, without really understanding the message conveyed by a person. Asking questions is the best way to get clarity and resolve all conflicts. Rather than getting angry, learn to communicate. Try NVC (non-violent communication), for example. Your world is not the world. It's just an interpretation of the world based on your past life. To enter the other person's world, it's important not to transfer your own world onto the other person. Just imagine: what if the other person had everything to teach us? Perhaps we would set aside our judgements and simply be present and listen.

4 - Always do your best
Whatever the circumstances, the context, your state of being, tell me sincerely if you're not always doing your best. If not, it's because your current life is too far removed from who you are. If not, simply acknowledge it! Stop trying to be perfect. Excellence is achieved through this simple intention: to be persevering by always doing your best. So always do your best, no more, no less.

Post these four rules for living that help to reframe the mind and align it with our soul.

- **Third Exercise: Regularly reset your habits**

We are creatures of habit. Routines make us feel secure, but in the long run they also make us rigid. And do you know why? Because we want to do more and more. In the end, we have the feeling that time is running away from us because we're in a frantic race. Like a mouse in a little wheel, spinning and doing the same thing over and over again. That's why we're going to develop our mental flexibility!

Of course, habits allow us to make repetitive gestures that give us control over what we do. A film that epitomises this idea is Charlie Chaplin's Modern Times. But the truth is, it's like always driving on the motorway. Our brain will always use the same lane, the same neural circuit. The danger is that, in the long run, we no longer manage to change our habits because we start to fear changing lanes. Normal, our brain has eliminated all the neural pathways we no longer use to reinforce the main one. If you change your habits, new neuronal channels will be created. At first, you'll have the impression that you're going backwards, that you're stalling, that you're not doing well enough. That's OK! Leave yourself alone and let your brain do its work.

Changing your habits is part of changing your life. So let's get started! Change the position of your bed, your sofa, your place at the table. When you go to work, take a different route from time to time. Arrange the things on your desk differently. Go and work in a café. Go away for the weekend at the last minute, eat in a restaurant with unfamiliar flavours and dishes. Read an incomprehensible book, dance to unfamiliar rhythms, sing, walk in a novel way. Complacency is the enemy of the good if we are not fully satisfied with our lives.

On the other hand, when we are in habits that are healthy for us, i.e. that allow us to be serene and fully fulfilled, i.e. that the body-soul-mind are in the same alignment, then it will be possible to maintain these new habits while continuing to maintain mental flexibility. Our brain is a muscle that adapts to our life. If your life doesn't suit you, you know what to do: change your habits.

3. The little door of the mind: from individual consciousness to universality

But who runs the computer? And what powers this computer? It's what we call the Universal Spirit, universal consciousness, full presence, God, Allah, the great 'all', energy, the great architect, the power of intention... It is a field of emptiness that contains all creation outside space and time. This universe is vibratory, energy and pure consciousness. To simplify understanding, I'll use the words GOD or INTENTION, which are, according to my vision, what I use on a daily basis. I invite you, if this doesn't speak to you, to replace these words with the one that resonates most with you.

If you do not believe in the existence of GOD, I invite you to read the book "DIEU, la science, les preuves" by Michel-Yves Bolloré and Olivier Bonnassies, which might open your conscience to a more pragmatic and scientifically proven vision of this truth... As I am not here to debate this subject, I apologise in advance for my very sketchy vision, as nothing can rationalise the existence of GOD, who is omnipotent, omnipresent and omniscient.

According to certain religious movements, it is written in ancient texts that God shaped the world, from light to man. But man is still only a creature; God is all-powerful, unique and an actor. So he withdraws, withholding his power so that the world may be and man may enter history. God renounces his omnipresence and leaves room for Creation to exist. In this way, he leaves man free to choose... even if he decides to reject him and choose the path of darkness.

By withdrawing, it has allowed the soul to create its own universe in conjunction with the mind, but when we were born we forgot our link to GOD. The human body is what enables us to experience this creation and the mind to understand its mechanisms. It is through this empty space that we have been able to create the world we contemplate every moment through our senses. So God has withdrawn, but at any moment we can ask him to come back and live a divine experience.

Our senses encourage our identification with the body through the mind, which is a reproduction of the universal spirit (the macrocosm) in a body (the microcosm). Otherwise we would only be spirit and therefore GOD. If we are the creator, it is impossible to recognise and identify ourselves as a being because we are 'everything'. How can a computer know that it is a computer? Because it identifies with what the creator has said about it, that it is a computer. It has therefore withdrawn to allow the soul and the mind to create the story of our existence by identifying ourselves with this world, which is what we call illusion. And which for all of us is reality. This is why certain schools of thought say that this world is an illusion created by our soul and our mind (the sacred couple) and that the real truth is found only within us, in GOD.

But GOD is what makes up the "whole". If our soul does not recognise GOD or this universal consciousness in everything, then we will feel an "anxious emptiness" and sometimes even an abyss of suffering.

The emptiness that is an interpretation of the mind is really the cause of our primordial fear, the fear of the soul that is estranged from its source. The fear that led us to this feeling of separation, the cause of all our ills.

On the other hand, GOD or full presence is the source of all feelings of bliss, happiness, serenity and inner peace. When we connect with this universal consciousness, a powerful inner silence floods over us and takes us out of the time-space of the world of illusions. All our problems and ills vanish. This is what makes the miracle possible. Because a miracle is a connection to a space of emptiness (GOD) which is at the origin of transcendental creation. Since illness no longer exists in this space-time, it simply disappears like our problems, hence the word miracle to shed light on these unexplained cures.

In short, it is through this uncreated (GOD withdrawing from creation) that evil (or the absence of good, of consciousness) arises and conversely good, which is a law of polarities according to Hermetic principles. An inner separation is created, a deep breach in which all our evils will appear. Justice then appears with its laws and obligations to restore harmony. Without justice and balance, our bodies tip over into mental or physical suffering.

The only way to heal ourselves is to accept to replace this emptiness and this belief that unconsciously terrifies us by welcoming the existence of the divine within us. It is then that we can access the pearl, the alchemists' treasure, the gold, the radiance, the genie in the lamp, absolute truth, ultimate liberation, total faith, wholeness, nirvana.

The universal spirit is therefore an energy and a higher consciousness, but also a set of vibrations that can be found on ten planes of consciousness.

Universal consciousness is symbolised by the colour black. It is full presence. It is the original matrix that integrates the essence of the universe and creation, nothingness and everything, the ain soph for the Kabbalists, the alpha and the omega, the beginning and the end. The associated mathematical number is zero. The vibration is 174 hertz.

The white chakra of the star of the earth is linked to birth. It is the primordial light, absolute unity, the union of soul and matter, the origin of life on earth, the ain soph aur for Kabbalists. The number is one. The vibration is 285 hertz.

The red root chakra is linked to our incarnation and the spirit of life. It is our foundation, the base of our spine and what allows us to feel safe, active and centred. The number is two. The vibration is 396 hertz in the Sacred Solfeggio (SS) and 342 hertz on the Electromagnetic Frequencies of Colours (FEC), and the associated note is C.

The orange sacral chakra is linked to creativity and the spirit of holiness. It is the home of the "I" and the centre of our sexuality. It governs our relationship to pleasure, abundance and well-being in our lives. The number is three. The vibration is 417 hertz for the SS and 480 hertz for the FEC, and the note is D.

The yellow solar plexus chakra is linked to beauty and power. It is the control centre of the will, of self-acceptance and self-esteem and of the meaning given to our values. The number is four. The vibration is 528 hertz for the SS and the same for the FEC, and the note is E.

The green heart chakra is linked to love and compassion. It governs emotional healing. It is the control centre for our relationship with ourselves and others, i.e. the spiritual and material worlds. The number is five. The vibration is 639 hertz for the SS and 594 hertz for the FEC, and the note is F.

The sky-blue throat chakra is linked to speech and the spirit of truth. It is the centre of communication, responsibility, faith and listening. It allows us to manifest positive situations in our lives when we express ourselves with love. The number is five. The vibration is 741 hertz for the SS and 672 hertz for the FEC, and the note is G.

The indigo third eye chakra is linked to intuition and strength. It develops our intellectual capacities and enlightens our perceptions. It expands our psychic abilities and our consciousness, and gives us access to a spirit of wisdom. The number is six. The vibration is 852 hertz for the SS and 720 hertz for the FEC, and the note is LA.

The violet coronal chakra is linked to receptivity and the spirit of sacrifice. It is the control centre for our connection to our soul mission, our purpose and the vision of our future. The number is seven. The vibration is 963 hertz for the SS and 768 hertz for the FEC, and the note is SI.

The golden chakra of the higher soul or star gate is linked to ascension and the eternal spirit. It is symbolised by the chalice, the receptacle that unifies the human and the divine and gives access to an innate knowledge of the soul. It is access to a higher consciousness where we can feel and experience divine love. The number is eight. The vibration is the perfect harmonic of all the vibrations in our different energy bodies.

The divine or universal spirit chakra allows you to connect directly to the source. This activation connects you to the flow of spirit and enables you to live in divine grace. It's a surrender to life and a detachment from the grip of matter. It enables us to live in the eternal present. It is the activation of the divine and the spiritual body in matter. The number is nine. It is the end of a cycle before beginning a new cycle of life.

When we explore these ten levels of consciousness and refine them over the course of our lives, we nourish our being with the spirit of GOD. This will reveal within us access to extrasensory perceptions such as clairaudience, clairvoyance, clairsentience, telepathy, claircognition, etc., which are simply innate multipotentials to which everyone has access.

To develop these different multi-potentialities, we need to be aware that we don't know anything. That what we think we know is wrong. That this world is an illusion and that reality is within us, within GOD. Because only the humble of spirit can open the small door that will lead them to a divine life. The ego cannot enter this sacred space, because accepting that you have been completely wrong about your life requires a great deal of courage and vulnerability. Recognising that we know nothing about ourselves is the first step towards transforming our lives.

It is then that in the philosophical current, we will go through the path of virtues. In alchemy, we go to the crucible to transform lead into gold and reveal the philosopher's stone. In the Christian religion, we struggle against sin and fight against Leviathan (the devil or dragon) to become Christ. In shamanism, we connect to the sacred with a loving intention to heal our being and be fully connected to the greater whole. In ancient Egypt, we go through initiation to learn how to master our vibratory levels. In today's science, we seek to discover the origin of the universe and try to prove the existence of the singularity that created our solar system, the big bang. Whatever path we take, or even if we take them all and more, we thirst for spirituality, we thirst to meet ourselves in our wholeness and our unity. We thirst for love, for returning to the source of our Being, for experiencing the divine within ourselves.

There's no one path that's better than another; I've discovered that each one opens up my consciousness. Each one brings a key. Being open to the world is the first key. To believe that you know everything is to close the door on yourself, or rather "self-love".

Patience will then be required, as the path may seem long and tedious. The more fluidly we embrace change and listen to ourselves, the faster the path. That's why the preceding stages are essential to prepare you for your growth.

The following exercises are fundamental foundations that really help to bring about an inner revolution and a concrete connection to the self. But it's in the journey and the action that you'll understand the secrets.

3.1 Practical exercises

- **First exercise: the power of intention**

GOD is therefore a mysterious force that structures the universe and acts as its creator. We all have this creative force within us, but we use it to a limited extent because of our beliefs and mental programmes. This is why I will be drawing on the vision of Dr Wayne W. DYER and his book *"The Power of Intention"* to help us connect with the divine and open that little door.

To this end, Dr Wayne W. Dyer presents seven faces of Intention to cultivate in our daily lives, offering different perspectives for understanding and integrating this concept into our lives and becoming a wiser, more mature being:

1. **Creativity:** Intention is a fundamental creative force in the universe. By recognising our capacity to be co-creators of our world, we can channel this creative energy into manifesting our deepest desires.
2. **Kindness:** the intention is intrinsically benevolent. By aligning our actions and thoughts with this intention of

kindness, we can cultivate harmonious relationships and make a positive contribution to the world around us.

3. **Love:** intention is fundamentally 'love'. By opening ourselves up to unconditional love, we can connect with universal intention and create a life filled with compassion, joy and harmony.
4. **Beauty:** intention seeks to guide us towards what is beautiful and authentic in our lives. By appreciating the beauty around us and seeking to create beauty in our actions, we can live a more fulfilling and rewarding life.
5. **Abundance:** intention is an abundant force that seeks to provide us with everything we need to flourish. By adopting an abundance mentality and practising gratitude, we can attract more wealth into our lives.
6. **Expansion:** Intention is an expansive force that seeks to guide us towards our full potential. By opening our minds and embracing new possibilities, we allow intention to lead us towards personal growth and fulfilment.
7. **Receptivity:** intention needs to be listened to and followed. By being receptive to the signs and indications of intention, we can align ourselves with our true path and live a life more in line with our deepest desires.

By integrating these seven faces of intention into our daily lives, we can create a reality more aligned with our highest aspirations and live a life of happiness, peace and self-fulfilment.

Here's a practical exercise inspired by the book "The Power of Intention". by Dr Wayne W. Dyer:

Find a quiet place: look for a quiet space where you can relax and concentrate without being disturbed.

Centre yourself with your breathing: sit comfortably with your back straight. Close your eyes and take a few deep breaths to relax. Pay attention to your breathing, feeling the air flowing in and out of your lungs.

Clarify your intention: think about a clear, positive intention that you want to manifest in your life. This intention can concern any aspect of your life, whether it's your health, your relationships, your career or your personal development.

Visualise your intention being realised: by concentrating on your breathing, start to visualise your intention as if it had already been realised. Imagine yourself living the reality of your intention with all your senses. Feel the positive emotions associated with achieving your goal.

Cultivate a feeling of gratitude: express gratitude for the realisation of your intention, as if it were already a reality. Thank the universe, your higher self or any other force that you believe can help you manifest your intention.

Let go: Once you've clarified your intention and cultivated a sense of gratitude, let go of the outcome. Trust the processes of the universe and be open to the possibilities and synchronicities that may come your way.

Take inspired action: remain attentive to the signs and indications of the universe, and be ready to take inspired action to manifest your intention in the real world. Follow your intuition and act in line with your intention.

Practise regularly: repeat this exercise regularly to strengthen your intention and maintain a deep connection with your goals. The more you practise this visualisation, the more you'll strengthen your ability to manifest your desires in your life.

By practising this exercise regularly, you can cultivate the power of intention and begin to create the life you truly desire.

- **Second exercise – Energy cleansing, anointing and prayer**

In this section, we explore a more global vision of being. Responding to unconscious needs is necessary to purify our soul-mind relationship and cleanse our energy bodies.

The first is the bowl of hot water, a practice as old as the hills. The aim is to cleanse our bodies by creating a sweating effect. The high vibration of the heat encourages the elimination of toxins and promotes the body's energetic circulation. I invite you to drink a large bowl of the hottest water possible every morning (without burning yourself), thinking about your intentions for the day.

The second is the Scottish shower or cold shower. Switching from hot to cold promotes the vibratory cleansing of our different bodies, because what distinguishes hot from cold is a change in vibratory levels. Hot detoxifies, while cold strengthens and firms. Starting with warmth is therefore a good way of extracting toxins, opening the skin's pores, cleansing and then closing them. It's very important to use healthy products on the skin to avoid clogging the pores, which need to breathe in order to oxygenate the whole body. The skin absorbs what you put on it, so take great care of it. You can also imagine that the water flowing over your body has the power to cleanse you in every dimension of your being.

A hot bath or, if you don't have a bath, a foot bath with coarse salt once a week is an excellent way to cleanse yourself energetically. When we've had a stressful week, and we've been around people who are in a bad frame of mind, grumbling or suffering, there's nothing better than a good bath to cleanse all that away. A few candles and essential oils can be used to help you relax. The best thing is to do it as a ritual before starting your weekend. You'll then be able to make the most of your time off.

Incense and fumigation with white sage, for example, have been used since the dawn of time to cleanse rooms and practitioners. Smoke gives you access to all the spaces in a room. When you're around an unpleasant person, you may have the feeling that you're still carrying that person's energy around with you. So, I invite you to take some incense or sage and imagine that the smoke is purifying you in the same way that fire cleanses a space. Set the intention you wish to replace the one you were wearing. You'll see, it's magical.

Anointing is a way of bringing us back to gentleness by rubbing oil on our bodies or going for a massage. It's about feeling the universe, the air, the touch on our skin. It means letting ourselves be touched and opening up to the world by letting our shell melt away. How many people are really aware of this moment in the morning when we put cream on our face? It's important to take a moment with ourselves where we bring that softness that is so fundamental to our lives. How many people suffer from a lack of caresses, a lack of gentleness... Why do we always want it to come from outside? What if everything started with you? Emotional autonomy begins with small gestures that become natural. Give yourself a gentle, enveloping massage once in a while – it feels so good. How many people have never had a massage in their lives? It's frightening. It makes no sense to want to take care of others without doing it for yourself.

Prayer is a sacred moment of communion with GOD, just like our intentions or any connection to our spirituality. It is an act, codified or not, that we can practise at home and at any time. Giving thanks could be considered an act of prayer. This moment can really change your life. Praying means keeping hope alive for a better world. It's about being able to communicate with all parts of ourselves in all our dimensions. It's about having faith in life and love. It's a moment of connection with the greater whole. It's a moment of silence with ourselves. It's also about expressing what's bothering us and our anger without offending anyone, so that we can make peace with ourselves.

- **Third exercise – Revealing your inner guidance through automatic writing**

So this is a little-known activity, isn't it? And yet it's a very good way of putting our feelings on paper. That's why you need a quiet space, a diary and a pen to practise this method. Writing down everything that comes into your head every day is a way of freeing your mind. Sometimes, without realising it, we go over and over things in our minds. Seeing them transcribed on paper gives us the material to obtain solutions, answers to get us out of unsolvable situations or problems. But how is it that we then find the solution? It's up to you to answer this question. Try it, it's brilliant!

- **Fourth exercise – Liberating forgiveness**

Forgiveness is a voluntary act whereby a person decides to let go of feelings of resentment, anger or resentment towards another person who has wronged them, even if that person has not necessarily expressed remorse or apologised. It is an emotional and psychological process that enables the injured person to free themselves from the emotional burden associated with the injury or injustice they have suffered.

Forgiveness does not necessarily mean forgetting or minimising the seriousness of what happened, or justifying or excusing the behaviour of the person responsible. On the contrary, it is a way for the person who has been hurt to regain control of their emotions and their life, and to heal and rebuild after being hurt.

Forgiveness can bring many benefits to the forgiver, including reduced stress, anxiety and anger, improved mental and physical health, increased empathy and compassion, and restored interpersonal relationships.

It is important to note that forgiveness is a personal process that can take time and should not be imposed or rushed. Everyone moves towards forgiveness at their own pace, and it is sometimes necessary to call on professional support or additional resources to achieve this.

Forgiveness has the power to transform our lives in miraculous ways. So, start by forgiving the little things. And one day you'll be the embodiment of peace and true love.

- **Fifth exercise – Listening to sacred music**

"If you want to find the secrets of the universe, think in terms of energy, frequency, information and vibration." Nicolas Tesla

This is why certain specific frequencies mentioned above can be a real stimulant in your daily life, at work, in the car or before going to bed. It's a solfeggio that was used in Gregorian chants and had the power to heal and harmonise the vibrations of the physical and energetic bodies.

The frequencies seen above through our different energy bodies have their own rhythms, their own vibrations. You can find them on YouTube according to your own aspirations.

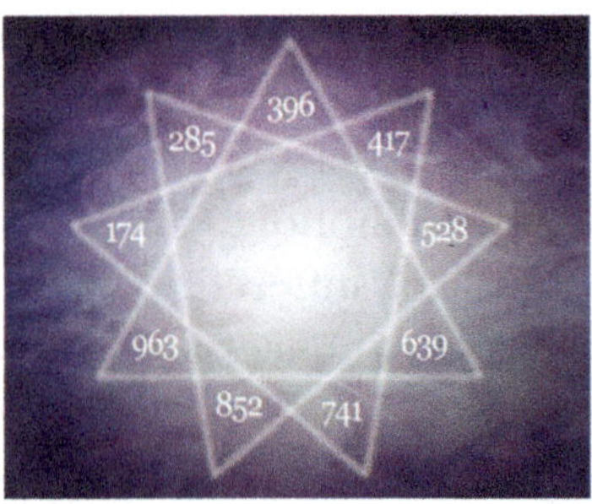

The sounds and people we listen to have a huge impact on our lives. When we rest on the banks of a stream, our mind calms down and our emotions melt away with the current. Our overall energy is balanced and we return home in peace. The sounds emitted act on our own frequencies, harmonising or unbalancing them. If we listen to anxiety-provoking news on television, this directly disturbs the frequencies of our root chakra and we unconsciously feel an inner sense of insecurity if we validate this bad news. This leads us to lose confidence in life. Take care to surround yourself with good vibes. Aggressive music and people giving off bad vibes disrupt your energy.

CHAPTER 17

Key remedies for health

Biotherapies during the dry fasting cure

1. The benefits of walking

Walking is useful because the body expends less energy when walking than when sitting or standing. This is because a person moves like a pendulum, transferring the weight of the body from one foot to the other. For the body, this is more natural and easier compared with the energy costs involved in keeping the body in a fixed vertical state. What's more, walking is useful because every muscle is working. Even the smallest muscle says *"I'm moving, that means I'm alive"*, because movement is life. We live thanks to the movement of our muscles. We look and our eye muscles contract, we move and every muscle in the body works. Even the heart is just a muscle. As long as this main muscle is working, we are alive. When walking, the body moves the legs simultaneously in three planes: vertical, longitudinal and transverse. The faster the walking rhythm, the greater the amplitude of vertical movements, the more active the muscular and linking systems and the more intense the energy expenditure. Working the legs activates blood circulation. The blood intensely enriches the internal organs with oxygen and speeds up metabolic processes. Regular walks in the fresh air boost health and improve well-being.

The respiratory, muscular and cardiovascular systems are strengthened. Muscular activity improves blood flow in the veins. The therapeutic benefits are the prevention of varicose veins and the elimination of toxins from the body. In addition, active energy processes eliminate fat: 15 minutes at an average pace (1.5 km) burns 100 kcal. The benefits of walking for men are due to the fact that stagnant processes in the pelvic area are eliminated. Walking also helps to prevent somatic diseases, hypodynamia and musculoskeletal disorders. Regular walking improves immunity and stamina, has a positive effect on mental health and improves sleep.

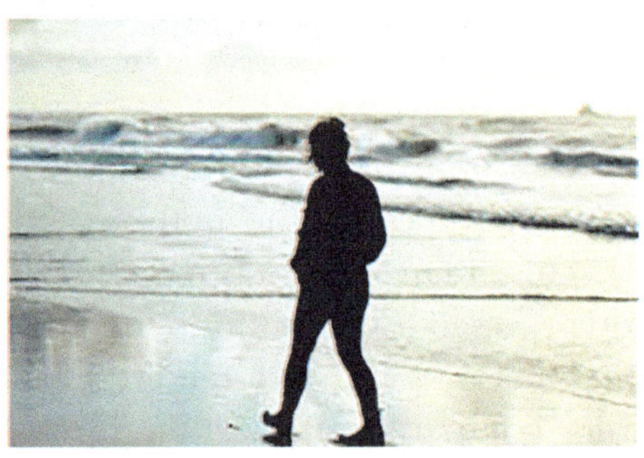

Walking is good for the spine because the vertebrae are strengthened and massaged as they take their place while walking. Blood starts to flow, even to hard-to-reach places, and the rocking of the vertebrae creates a massage effect. The supply to the intervertebral discs is perfectly improved. The chondrocytes only receive nourishment during calm movements, so protrusions are treated. Therapeutic walking during protrusion is particularly useful for overweight people. Why is this? For them, it's a good opportunity to keep fit. Calm movements activate almost all the muscle groups. Walking is the best form of exercise for the spine, and no sport is as useful as walking. Therapeutic walking plays an important role in weight loss. You only need to devote an hour to this activity to burn around 30g of fat.

The benefits of walking are also seen in the work on the digestive system, as walking is an excellent massage for the internal organs. Walking barefoot and consciously is excellent because it provides a stimulating massage of all the organs underfoot. The benefits of walking are as follows.

1. **Improved mental health and emotional well-being**: Walking can significantly reduce symptoms of depression and anxiety. It offers a moment of relaxation and meditation, helping to clarify thoughts and reduce stress.
2. **Anti-ageing and longevity:** Studies have shown that regular walking can increase lifespan and slow down the ageing process. Walking improves cellular health and strengthens the immune system.
3. **Improving bone health and preventing osteoporosis**: Walking is a form of weight-bearing exercise that strengthens bones and increases bone density, thereby reducing the risk of fractures and osteoporosis, particularly in women after the menopause.
4. **Positive effects on cardiovascular health**: As well as strengthening the heart and reducing the risk of heart disease, regular walking can lower blood pressure and cholesterol, and improve blood circulation.
5. **Improved quality of sleep**: Regular walking can help to improve the quality of sleep, in particular by helping you to fall asleep more quickly and sleep more deeply.
6. **Increased lung capacity**: Walking increases lung capacity and improves respiratory efficiency, which is particularly beneficial for people suffering from chronic respiratory diseases.
7. **Positive effects on cognitive health**: Walking can improve cognitive function, strengthen memory and even reduce the risk of dementia and Alzheimer's disease.
8. **Improved balance and coordination**: Regular walking improves balance and coordination, reducing the risk of falls, particularly among the elderly.
9. **Socialising and connecting with nature:** Walking is often a social activity that allows you to connect with other people. Moreover, walking in green spaces or in nature offers

additional benefits linked to exposure to nature. This helps to improve mood and reduce stress.

Walking is useful because, when walking, the body expends less energy than when sitting or standing still. This is because a person moves like a pendulum, transferring the weight of the body from one foot to the other. For the body, this is more natural and easier than the energy costs associated with maintaining the body in a fixed vertical state. Walking is also useful because every muscle is working. Even the smallest muscle says "I'm moving, that means I'm alive", because movement is life. We live thanks to the movement of our muscles: we look and our eye muscles contract, we move and every muscle in the body works. Even the heart is just a muscle. As long as this main muscle is working, we are alive. When walking, the body moves the legs simultaneously in three planes: vertical, longitudinal and transverse. The faster the walking rhythm, the greater the amplitude of the vertical movements, the more active the muscular and linking systems and the more intense the energy expenditure. Working the legs while walking activates blood circulation and the blood intensely enriches the internal organs with oxygen, speeding up metabolic processes. Regular walks in the fresh air boost health and improve well-being.

The respiratory, muscular and cardiovascular systems are strengthened. Muscular activity improves blood flow in the veins. The result is the prevention of varicose veins and the elimination of toxins from the body. Active energy processes eliminate fat: 15 minutes walking at a moderate pace (1.5 km) burns 100 kcal.

The benefits of walking for men are due to the fact that stagnant processes in the pelvic region are eliminated. Walking is also beneficial in preventing somatic diseases, hypodynamia and musculoskeletal disorders. Regular walking improves immunity and stamina, has a positive effect on mental health and improves sleep.

First of all, walking is good for the spine: the vertebrae are strengthened and massaged, and take their place when you walk.

Blood starts to flow, even to hard-to-reach areas, and the rocking of the vertebrae creates a massage effect. The supply to the intervertebral discs is greatly improved. The chondrocytes only receive nourishment during calm movements, so protrusions are treated. Therapeutic walking during protrusion is particularly useful for overweight people. Why is this? For them, it's a good opportunity to keep fit. Calm movements activate almost all the muscle groups. Walking is the best exercise for the spine, and no sport is as useful as walking.

Walking therapy plays an important role in weight loss. You only need to devote an hour to this activity to burn around 30g of fat. Stable activities with health treatments will give you great pleasure with good results.

The benefits of walking can also be seen in the work on the digestive system, where there is an excellent massage of the internal organs. Walking barefoot and consciously is excellent and provides a stimulating massage of all the organs underfoot.

2. Ito thermie, the Japanese art of healing

Ito-Thermie combines the principles of five disciplines: acupuncture (actions on vital points), massage, moxibustion, aromatherapy and Shiatsu. Sticks of incense, made up of seven herbs (including pine, cedar, mugwort, Japanese medlar and keihi) and a mineral, are burnt in special metal instruments called reionki (冷温器). The reionki are then applied directly to the skin by means of a massage during a 15-20 minute session over the entire body, following a certain path or making circles or stopping at specific points (stop-points) as appropriate. It doesn't burn, quite the opposite: a sensation of softness and warmth invades the whole body as the session progresses.

- **Effects**

The massage and the heat transmitted by the incandescent incense sticks (infrared emission) generate profound effects:

these stimuli are absorbed by the body and used by all its vital functions. Ito-Thermie helps to restore balance to the autonomic nervous system by stimulating the immune, hormonal and digestive systems. The smoke from the incense is also beneficial thanks to its disinfectant and healing properties, which contribute to the virtuous effect of the technique as a whole. This discipline, which is widespread in Japan but still little-known in Europe, helps to relieve tension and relieve stress and fatigue. Its power and disconcerting effectiveness also make it an effective means of preventing illness.

General benefits

- All kinds of pain
- Allergies
- Infections
- Circulatory problems
- Insomnia
- Fertility problems
- Stress, depression
- Respiratory problems

- **Weak immunity and cancer**

Ito-Thermie also helps relieve muscle pain after sports training.

3. Fasciatherapy

Fasciatherapy is a gentle manual therapy method that focuses on the fascia, an essential component of the human body. Fascias are connective tissues that envelop and support all the organs, muscles, bones and nerves, forming a sort of continuous network throughout the body. This therapeutic approach aims to treat various physical and emotional dysfunctions by releasing tensions and restrictions within these tissues.

Fasciatherapy was developed in the 1970s by Danis Bois, a French physiotherapist and osteopath. Inspired by osteopathic techniques and psychosomatic research, fasciatherapy has evolved to incorporate a more holistic dimension to health, considering the interaction between body and mind.

The fundamental principle of fasciatherapy is based on the idea that fascia plays a crucial role in maintaining balance and health throughout the body. Tension, blockages or imbalances within this network can lead to pain, dysfunction and mobility problems. Fasciatherapy therefore seeks to:

- Release fascial restrictions to restore mobility and balance to the body.
- Stimulate the body's self-healing mechanisms.
- Improve circulation of body fluids.
- Promoting greater body awareness.

Fasciatherapy uses gentle manual techniques, which can vary according to the patient's specific needs. These techniques include gentle manipulation and stretching of the fascia to release tension and promote a state of deep relaxation. Some practitioners may also incorporate gentle movements and body awareness exercises to enhance the therapeutic effect.

Fasciatherapy is used to treat a wide range of problems:

- Musculoskeletal pain (back pain, neck pain, tendonitis, etc.)
- Mobility and musculoskeletal disorders
- Stress and stress-related disorders (anxiety, sleep disorders, etc.)
- Circulatory problems
- Digestive disorders

Patients who use fasciatherapy often report a significant improvement in their overall well-being, reduced pain, increased mobility, and a greater sense of relaxation and connection with their body. Fasciatherapy offers a holistic, non-invasive approach to treating a variety of physical and emotional problems. By focusing on the fascia, this therapeutic method seeks to restore balance and harmony to the body. As with any therapeutic intervention, it is advisable to consult a qualified professional to determine whether fascia therapy is suitable for your specific needs.

4. Oil pulling: a dry fasting preparation therapy using coconut oil

This detox method is very interesting and can also be used by people with health problems who don't want to do a dry fast. It disinfects the mouth and can improve any state of health. Three or five one-month cures a year is ideal. It can also be taken continuously. "Gandush", also known as "oil pulling", is a traditional Ayurvedic practice consisting of holding a spoonful of vegetable oil in the mouth for a few minutes in the morning. This 'detox' routine is reputed to have numerous benefits for oral health, while revitalising and purifying the body as a whole.

In Ayurveda, the age-old Indian medicine, 'gandouch', also known as 'kavala gandoosha' or 'kavala graha', is an essential oral hygiene ritual for waking up in the morning. Although the practice may seem simple, it can be confusing: it involves keeping a spoonful of sesame oil in the mouth for at least five minutes for novices and up to 20 minutes for regulars. It is recommended that the oil be circulated vigorously between the interstices of the teeth, from front to back. During this mouthwash, the oil is loaded with toxins, which are then expelled by spitting it out. When it comes into contact with the saliva, which acts as an emulsifier, the oil becomes cloudy and may take on a light colour, sometimes tending towards green.

For practical reasons, it is advisable not to spit the mixture down the sink to avoid clogging the drains. It's best to use a disposable tissue and dispose of it in a bin. Then rinse your mouth out with warm water and brush your teeth as usual. If necessary, use interdental floss and clean your teeth with a hose. This ritual is best performed on an empty stomach before breakfast. Before practising 'gandouch' in Ayurveda, tongue scraping with a copper scraper is often recommended.

According to Ayurvedic tradition, the benefits of 'gandouch' are numerous. It is said to promote better oral health, stronger, whiter teeth and fresh breath, and to soothe gum inflammation while reducing the risk of cavities. What's more, according to the Charaka Samhita, a fundamental text of Ayurveda, oil mouthwashes strengthen the jawbones and the voice, beautify the lips, improve the taste of food and purify speech. 'Gandush' is said to support the body by eliminating toxins known as 'ama' in Ayurveda, toxic residues resulting from incompletely digested substances that accumulate in the mouth and on the tongue overnight. It is also said to eliminate bacteria, viruses and pathogenic germs from the oral cavity, which is particularly important given the link established between oral hygiene and overall health.

Ultimately, adopting this routine requires personal experience, with a period of at least three weeks to potentially feel its effects. In the case of dental abscesses or gingivitis, adding tea tree essential oil to the oral oil may be beneficial. Finally, it is important to stress that 'gandouch' does not replace traditional tooth brushing, an essential step in oral hygiene.

- **Coconut oil pulling is a simple procedure.**

1. Before brushing your teeth, put a tablespoon of vegetable oil in your mouth.
2. Massage the oil into every corner of your mouth, moving your tongue vigorously and without swallowing the liquid. This process can take from ten to 20 minutes, depending on individual tolerance.
3. In the meantime, you can get on with other daily tasks such as making the bed, washing up or hanging out the washing. Taking care of other activities helps you forget about the discomfort of oil in your mouth.
4. After the allotted time, spit out the oil, rinse your mouth, brush your teeth as usual and that's it!

For optimum results, we recommend using coconut oil mouthwash at least once or twice a week, if not every day. In this case, the option of oil pulling with activated charcoal can be considered. Although the technique may seem strange at first, it will gradually become an unavoidable routine.

- **Why use oil pulling?**

Oil pulling is highly recommended because of the presence of various bacteria in the mouth, which can persist even with regular brushing. This method helps to effectively eliminate bacteria, contributing to whiter teeth and fresher breath.

- **What are the benefits of oil pulling?**

As well as whitening teeth and maintaining oral hygiene, oil pulling has positive effects on general health. By detoxifying the body, it provides energy and reduces inflammation (irritation, swollen gums), thanks to the oil's antibacterial and antibiotic properties.

- **When should I use oil pulling, in the morning or in the evening?**

Ideally, oil pulling is best done in the morning on an empty stomach, as no food has been eaten, making it easier to eliminate bacteria. However, if the morning is not convenient for you, this practice can also be carried out in the evening before bedtime.

- **Clinical study**

https://www.jpda.com.pk/wp-content/uploads/2018/06/01-ROLE-OF-COCONUT-OIL.pdf

5. Pucma therapeutic coverage

The therapeutic mechanism of the Pucma therapeutic blanket consists of reducing local convective heat loss from the body and reducing the intensity of the external effects of electromagnetic radiation. The results are the activation of the body's protective mechanisms, which have a positive effect on our health and resistance to disease and adverse environmental factors.

The therapeutic blanket consists of three layers: two outer and one inner. All the layers have a synthetic base. The difference lies in the fact that the inner layer consists of a metallic micron "screen" that serves to reflect electromagnetic radiation from our body. The outer surface of the therapeutic blanket acts as a sort of protective barrier against electromagnetic interference from the environment. The therapeutic blanket strengthens the body's resistance to disease and its harmful effects, reduces the frequency and severity of illness, relieves stress, cures depression and improves mood and work capacity.

Healing cover is used for:

- Safeguarding and strengthening health, boosting immunity;
- Preventing disease;
- Treating various diseases and disorders;
- Rehabilitating, revitalising and energising;
- Increasing the effectiveness of combined treatments;
- Reducing the side effects of medication;
- Reducing drug use, rehabilitating patients, the elderly, the disabled and patients with incurable diseases;
- Reducing the side effects of other treatment methods and synchronising biorhythms;
- Reducing vegetative and hormonal imbalances.

The cover was awarded the Paul Ehrich Medal by the European Academy of Clinical Immunology in Germany.

For the development of the *"method and device of multifactorial therapeutic action using multilayer therapeutic coverage"*, its author was awarded the Mechnikov Medal *"for his practical contribution to strengthening the nation's health"* by the Russian Academy of Natural Sciences. This non-pharmaceutical approach to restorative and corrective medicine aims to ensure effective recovery. It aims to prevent illness and relieve stress, depression and chronic fatigue. Therapeutic coverage transforms an initially unfavourable functional state of the human body into a more favourable one. This is achieved by optimising the functioning of the regulatory and protective sub-systems and improving the economy of the energy exchanges that essentially determine the state of health, the emotional and mental state, resistance to illness and stress, the severity of disorders and even the effectiveness of specific clinical treatments.

The complete wrap in the therapeutic blanket is used for rehabilitation, prevention and treatment of illnesses, including those caused by chronic stress. The procedure improves sleep, general well-being and mood, and increases resistance to stress factors.

Some areas of application:

- Prevention and treatment of respiratory organs: asthma, bronchitis, pneumonia, acute respiratory illnesses, acute respiratory viral infections, influenza.
- Diseases of the digestive system
- Kidney and urinary tract diseases, treatment of prostatitis, cystitis and pyelonephritis
- Prevention and treatment of osteoarthritis, arthritis and polyarthritis
- Osteochondrosis of the spine, sciatica (treatment and prophylaxis)
- Skin diseases
- Neuritis, neuralgia
- Prevention and treatment of neuroses, depression, chronic fatigue and insomnia.

Action factors

Wrapped in a blanket, thanks to the inner protective layer, the person is protected from external electrostatic and electromagnetic fields and our own energy (biofield) is able to redistribute itself throughout the body in the best possible way.

If there is a problem somewhere in the body, our own energy is directed towards the area in question to restore its functions. In the language of physiological processes, this means improving blood circulation and therefore metabolic processes, by initiating self-restoration mechanisms at hormonal, vegeto-vascular and other self-regulatory levels.

The sensations experienced under the blanket can vary from a hot flush to a tingling sensation in problem areas. But one thing remains constant: by using the blanket, the body begins to help itself. The most pronounced therapeutic effect is achieved following long-term treatment.

The product has won academic awards:

- Medal I. Mechnikov Medal of the Russian Academy of Natural Sciences
- P. Ehrlich Medal of the European Academy of Natural Sciences;
- Diploma in the competition "The best technology for diagnosing and improving health in regenerative medicine - 2003" of the Russian National Centre for Medical and Health Care of the Russian Ministry of Health.

Application of therapeutic cover:

The greatest therapeutic effect is achieved by a general wrap. The patient is wrapped in the blanket so that only their face remains exposed. When wrapping the patient in the blanket, the company emblem should be placed on the outside. The patient's underwear should contain a minimum of synthetic additives. Use a cotton blanket (duvet cover) to avoid dirt, damp and sweat. The patient should briefly touch an earthed object, such as a radiator, before the procedure. The procedures are carried out in a sitting or lying position, in a comfortable position, and the patient should relax as much as possible. The blanket is very relaxing and it is highly likely that the patient will fall asleep during the procedure.

The most common recommended course of treatment is ten to 14 days. If necessary, to increase efficacy and stabilise results, the course of treatment can be extended to 15-20 days. If necessary, courses of treatment should be repeated at intervals ranging from 14 days to one or two months. The cumulative therapeutic effect of the various interventions also means that the cure can have a prolonged effect, continuing after it has been completed. In some cases, the long-term results are even more favourable than immediately after treatment. In the treatment of chronic illnesses and the cure of serious diseases, the greatest effect is achieved through a series of procedures. This lasts six to eight procedures for some illnesses, eight to 12 for others, and more rarely 14 to 20 procedures.

To recover from a single stressful load, it is possible to carry out single sessions, i.e. to apply the blanket as and when required. The number of sessions per day depends on the objectives of the treatment. In addition to the full body wrap, it is recommended to combine the full body wrap with the partial body wrap or local application of the blanket when treating illnesses with pronounced local complaints. For local application, the product (in folded form) is applied to the site of the direct projection of the complaint (for example, on the projection of the pain). Start with ten minutes two or three times a day. Two times 20 minutes a day is ideal. Do not exceed 40 minutes per session. This therapy is part of our retreat group.

The product contains a special metallised film that creates the screen effect. It is fragile and must therefore be handled with care:

- steam method at a temperature of 110±2°C for 20-25 min;
- Air dry at 120±3°C for 45-50 minutes.

The product comes from Russia, so beware of copies from Europe. Sale of the product on the shop: www.jeunesec.com

6. Flower field acupressure mat, a friend for pain during fasting

We have a carpet on site but we recommend that you have your own to use in your room.

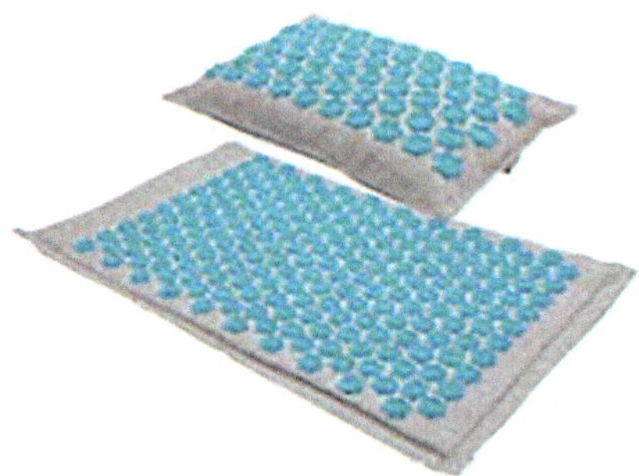

It's a thin acupressure mat, bristling with a multitude of tiny pimples. In the case of your Field of Flowers, 221 lotus flowers with 25 pointed petals are spread across the mat, making a total of more than 5,000 pimples. When you lie down with your back on the mat, the simple effect of your weight allows the pimples to act on your whole back at the same time.

This produces three reactions:

- Your body produces endorphins, which are pain-relieving hormones.
- The tension in your joints, muscles and nerves is released.
- Your blood circulation speeds up and your nervous system is stimulated.

The Champ de Fleurs mat is the result of a series of clinical tests which have shown it to be optimally effective: the results of the stimulation are enhanced and the sensation of discomfort caused by the spikes on the skin is greatly reduced. The spikes on the Champ de Fleurs mat do not penetrate the skin, and you can gradually get used to this sensation by starting to wear thin clothing. Regular use increases the benefits. Here's how a session works:

3 seconds: It stings! The nerves in the skin react to spikes. The first reaction is often to get up immediately.

1 minute: Blood begins to flow to the contact area of the lotus flower pimples.

2 minutes: A gentle sensation of warmth gradually replaces the tingling sensation.

5 minutes: The combination of heat and deep relaxation puts your body in a state of maximum relaxation.

10 minutes: At this point, muscle tension begins to release deeply.

30 minutes: Relieved of all pain and tension, it is common to fall asleep after a long session.

Here's what it does for your body:

- **Relaxation**
  - Works instantly on your body.
  - Soothes physical pain.
  - Calms and relieves inflammation.

- **Painkillers**
  - Generates endorphins.
  - Relaxes muscle tension.
  - Soothes nervous tension.

- **Regeneration**
  - Stimulates blood circulation.
  - Nourishes and moisturises the cells.
  - Brings oxygen to the cells.

- **Why use a Champ de Fleurs mat during dry fasting?**

1) Production of pain-relieving hormones

The nervous system is stimulated by the tiny spikes of lotus flowers scattered across the carpet. The body responds by producing endorphins, dopamine, serotonin and oxytocin, which are soothing and happy hormones. Thanks to their action, the nervous system no longer transmits pain. The pain is automatically soothed. These hormones have relaxing properties that help you get a good night's sleep: this is essential if the body is to find the resources to heal itself naturally. These hormones are never overdosed in your body, especially as it is the body itself that secretes them. They have beneficial effects in all cases. So there's no time limit for using a Champs de Fleur mat!

2) Soothing anddeep relaxation

The thousands of tiny pimples in the shape of lotus flowers stimulate your whole back at the same time, soothing your nervous system and relaxing your muscles. As a result, your back regains its flexibility and spinal agility. When you practise your Field of Flowers frequently, the whole body benefits.

3) A boost for the circulation

The smallest part of your back rests on the mat's small pimples. Arranged in the shape of little flowers, these pimples have been designed to stimulate the skin in the best possible way. This activates even the finest blood vessels to improve blood circulation. Better blood circulation means that oxygen and the vitamins and nutrients your body needs are better supplied. These elements reach the painful areas and help to heal and renew the cells in the best possible conditions.

The circulating blood brings what is needed to the cells, giving them the nourishment and hydration they need to renew themselves. It also removes toxins from the body. In this way, carbon dioxide is carried to the lungs to be expelled. The vertebrae also have constant exchanges with the blood, which provides them with water and oxygen. The vertebrae need a lot of water to remain mobile and function properly. The water supplied by the blood enables them to retain all their faculties. So good blood circulation is vital for the health of your back, and your health in general.

- **Little flower-shaped spikes**

All the devices are designed to offer maximum efficiency while promoting well-being. The design of the lotus flowers is not just a question of style! They allow every bit of skin to be stimulated as it rests on them, activating the meridians. Lying on a spiked mat is in fact a very comfortable and subtle way of looking after your health, as it stimulates well-being hormones such as endorphin.

For optimum results, we recommend that you lie on the mat for between a quarter of an hour and three-quarters of an hour, so that the pain-relieving effect can unfold gradually. It's over time that the body triggers an effective reaction and receives the most benefits.

The pimples contain no products that are harmful to your skin. They have been carefully designed and manufactured in Europe using ultra-precise moulding techniques. They are made from HIPS plastic, which is also recommended for food use, and rubber, which gives them the ideal flexibility to retain their corolla shape while acting precisely on your back. All these choices combine to create an effective, long-lasting device.

Soon enough, you won't need this garment any more and you'll appreciate the sensation of your Field of Flowers next to your skin. The effects mentioned above, the release of endorphins and improved blood circulation, will give you a feeling of well-being and pleasant warmth.

There are no strict instructions about the time and regularity of use of a Champ de Fleurs mat. But it is recommended that you lie down for at least 15 minutes for the benefits to be felt, and up to 45 minutes if you feel the need. Ideally, regular use will maximise the benefits: we recommend frequent or even daily use, to maximise the effects over time. But it is also possible to use the Flower Field occasionally, when a specific pain occurs. If setting aside a specific period of time to lie on the acupressure mat seems too restrictive, you can try lying on it in the evening before going to bed or in the morning before getting up.

- **Scientific research**

The design of the Champ de Fleurs acupressure mat is protected by a patent. It is the result of extensive research to obtain precise and effective results. It is perfectly designed to maximise pain relief, blood stimulation, and nerve and muscle relaxation, whatever the person using it. As soon as it was launched, Champ de Fleurs won over its users and proved its effectiveness to the general public. It is thanks to word of mouth from satisfied customers that the mat has been so successful in France. The University of Latvia, within the European Union, has been the centre of research and has been able to prove, through highly supervised tests, the therapeutic benefits that we cite here: its pain-relieving effect, its propensity to improve blood circulation and oxygen supply throughout the body, the diffusion of endorphins, and the benefits for energy and sleep.

- **The Champ de Fleurs cushion, belt and leg set**

Where the body becomes rounder, whether in the curves of the spine, in the lumbar and cervical regions, or in the bend of the knee, the use of the acupressure cushion will ideally complement the Champ de Fleurs mat. When lying down, an even larger surface area will be stimulated at once by the acupressure pimples. Adding one or two cushions to your mat will optimise the effects of this method.

Next, the area specially targeted by the Champ de Fleurs belt is the lumbar area. This part of the back is subject to a lot of strain in everyday life and requires special care. Targeted acupressure relaxes muscles and joints, stimulates blood circulation and releases pain-relieving hormones, oxytocins and endorphins. What's more, wearing the acupressure belt has a lasting effect, helping to support the back by stimulating the deep muscles that keep the back straight. It's up to you to adjust the strength of the action of your lumbar belt. You can choose a light effect by leaving the belt a little slack or a powerful action by tightening the belt around you. This one-size-fits-all belt is suitable for most body shapes, up to a maximum waist circumference of 120cm.

In addition to the devices already mentioned, mats, cushions or lumbar belt, you can further enhance the sensations of well-being and therapeutic effects of the Champ de Fleurs range by also stimulating your legs. Use the same acupressure method by wrapping the Champ de Fleurs leg set around your legs. The result is both a local effect on the newly stimulated areas, and a general effect, potentiating the effects on the whole body. It should be noted that the effect of the Champ de Fleurs leg set does not stop at the legs, but can help to relieve the pain felt in the back. In fact, all these parts of the body are linked and interact: relaxed legs help to relieve a back that is too tense, and the relief of sciatica or cruralgia extends to the lower back. Gaining mobility in the lower limbs also improves mobility in the lumbar area. Finally, the benefits in terms of blood circulation and the secretion of endorphins are of course felt throughout the body, whatever the area stimulated.

The acupressive method is effective on all areas of the body. Adding stimulation of the legs to classic stimulation of the back amplifies the beneficial effects of this method in all areas:

- Quality of sleep: the soothing effects of acupressure will be multiplied by extending the area of acupressure stimulation.
- Reducing stress: the back is the primary target of the effects of stress. But the legs also accumulate tension. It's a large area of skin, rich in nerve endings, which we sometimes forget about, and which deserves care and attention.

What's more, the effect of the pimples on the skin dynamically stimulates the nervous system, bringing it back into balance and helping to alleviate typical nerve pain in the legs, such as sciatica and cruralgia.

- **Soothing muscles**

Thanks to improved blood circulation and a more responsive nervous system, muscles also benefit from acupressure. When they have been overworked or even damaged, muscles need rest and increased blood flow to obtain the oxygen and nutrients they need to repair themselves. Whether you're suffering from cramps or even contractures and strains, acupressure will help your body regenerate. Similarly, joint pain such as tendonitis or osteoarthritis will be alleviated thanks to the improved functioning of the blood and nervous systems. The leg set consists of two parts that can be used on the same leg at different heights, or on the same area with both legs at the same time. To cover the surface of both legs, you will need to buy two Champ de Fleurs leg sets.

7. The benefits of dry brushing: do it yourself

- **Skin detoxification**

Dry brushing is a genuine beauty ritual, and its benefits are well established. Dry brushing is a beauty ritual in which a body brush is used on the skin without water or products. The brush is brushed over the body dry. One of the main benefits of dry brushing is that it deeply cleanses the skin, ridding it of all impurities. Dry brushing also stimulates lymphatic and blood circulation, leaving the skin soft, healthy and more toned. By boosting circulation, bodily waste products are better eliminated, preventing illness and infection.

- **Cellulite reduction**

Detoxifying the skin removes toxins. And unfortunately it's these toxins and water retention that cause cellulite. Thanks to the benefits of dry brushing, this orange-peel effect is less noticeable. Fatty deposits are reduced by dry brushing and are better distributed.

- **Improved blood circulation**

As with lymphatic circulation, another benefit of dry brushing is improved blood circulation. The body's waste products are eliminated much more effectively thanks to better oxygenation of the cells and a recharge of nutrients. By improving blood circulation, swelling, varicose veins and cellulite are reduced.

- **Gentle exfoliation**

With its rotating movements and brisk brushing action, one of the first benefits of dry brushing is that it gently exfoliates the skin. Once dead skin cells have been removed, cell regeneration can take place. Dry brushing makes the skin softer and more radiant, and also helps it to absorb skincare products more easily.

- **A feeling of well-being**

The final, and by no means least, benefit of dry brushing is the sense of well-being it brings. Relaxing, it's an anti-stress treatment that releases tension.

- **Enhancing the benefits of dry brushing**

To get the most out of dry brushing, you need to choose the right brush. Choose a brush with natural, relatively soft bristles. It should be cleaned with soap, without soaking. And to enhance the benefits of dry brushing, it's important to adopt the right technique. You should use circular strokes, starting at the ends of the limbs and working your way up towards the heart. To maximise the benefits of dry brushing, you should proceed as follows and in order:

- Brush under the feet, then over the top
- Move up the legs in circular movements
- Massage your hands, then apply the brush to your back
- Brush the buttocks using circular movements
- Finish with the stomach and chest, using gentler movements
- Take a cold shower to promote blood circulation
- Dry brushing can be carried out every day for ten to 15 minutes.

8. Tips to improve blood and lymph circulation before and after dry fasting

1. Draining phytotherapy

Here is a selection of plants known for their benefits on blood and lymph circulation.

- **Nettle:** Rich in flavonoids and minerals, it is known as a depurative and diuretic. It remineralises the body and helps to eliminate toxins that accumulate in the body.
- **Meadowsweet**: Rich in flavonoids, toning and draining, it improves blood circulation and helps eliminate water and toxins.
- **Dandelion leaves**: Known as an exceptional diuretic plant, they are effective in reducing water retention and promoting detoxification. Prepare the mixture in a herbalist's shop or with Quantis in equal parts. One teaspoon before meals in a little water.

1. Quantis two vials.

Equal parts nettle, meadowsweet and dandelion. www.LPEV.fr
For Swiss nationals, free number: 0800563382
For Belgians, free number 080071098
For the French: +33470906145
If you are asked for a practitioner number, give this one 1490664

Not all plants are suitable for pregnant or breast-feeding women, so always ask your doctor for advice.

9. Massages with essential oils and vegetable oils

Apply and massage until absorbed, so that the oils penetrate all the layers of the epidermis. Ideally, when the skin is still damp after a shower, for better absorption! If you're having beauty salon treatments, ask your specialist to use your own oil with natural draining properties! You can add two essential oils to vegetable oil. You can choose between vetiver, Italian helichrysum, mastic pistachio or cypress. The dosage is 10% essential oils to 90% vegetable oil.

10. Cold water jets after a shower

Cold water has a vasoconstrictive effect that increases blood pressure by constricting the blood vessels. In the shower or when you get out of the bath, run a jet of cold water from your ankles to the top of your thighs, working upwards.

11. Lymphatic drainage

This is a very gentle massage, to be carried out by a qualified therapist, which stimulates lymph circulation and helps to eliminate various waste products via the lymphatic channels. Several sessions are required, and it's a treatment that can be done all year round to stimulate the body.

12. Keep sufficiently hydrated

Remember to keep well hydrated every day! It's advisable to drink about 1.5 litres of water a day, which is equivalent to about ten glasses of water. If you have cellulite or water retention, it's essential to improve blood and lymph circulation to help your body eliminate toxins. You can use www.Marah.ch brand magnets that can be left in the water to improve drainage.

13. Suitable cuts of clothing and textiles

One of the main factors hindering the circulation of blood and lymph is the choice of clothes that are too tight, compressing the body and encouraging the accumulation of cellulite. Ideally, especially in summer, you should wear looser-fitting clothes made from natural materials such as cotton, silk, linen, etc. Don't forget that the body needs to breathe!

14. Salmanoff bath

Salmanoff baths, using hot water and turpentine, are renowned for their many health benefits, tested and documented by Dr Alexandre Salmanoff. They are particularly effective for:

- Improving blood and capillary circulation, including in areas with insufficient microcirculation, which is beneficial for cardiovascular and vascular diseases, and venous insufficiency.
- Stimulating metabolism in the nervous system and muscle tissue, which is useful for osteoarticular diseases, joint pain and spinal pathologies.
- Preventing and treating the severe complications of diabetes, by improving diabetic angiopathy and accelerating tissue healing.
- Helping treat skin problems such as furunculosis, psoriasis and scleroderma by accelerating healing and promoting skin rejuvenation.
- Contributing to weight loss and cellulite reduction by improving microcirculation and normalising lipid metabolism.

These baths are also recommended for their relaxing and detoxifying effects, encouraging perspiration and helping to eliminate toxins from the body. They are performed following specific procedures regarding water temperature and bath duration, and can be complemented by the addition of natural substances such as clay, seaweed or sea salt to enhance their beneficial effects.

However, there are some contraindications, particularly for people with certain heart conditions, people with severe asthenia or pregnant women. It is therefore advisable to consult a health professional before beginning a Salmanoff bath cure.

15. Baking soda cure

In warm water. Cures for a maximum of one month, twice a year. One teaspoon once or twice a day in a little warm water. Baking soda, when added to lukewarm water, offers a variety of health benefits, due to its antiseptic, alkalinising and anti-inflammatory properties. However, it is important to note that there is no solid scientific evidence to support the effectiveness of baking soda as a specific blood cleansing treatment or as an anti-cancer treatment. Here are some of the benefits generally associated with drinking baking soda water, based on traditional uses:

- **Antiseptic effect:** Baking soda can help eliminate viruses and bacteria that cause illness, thanks to its mild antiseptic effect. It is used to relieve sore and inflamed throats by gargling.

It acts as a blood cleanser and mild blood thinner, making it useful before a dry fast.

- **Relief from urinary tract infections:** By reducing the acidity of urine, bicarbonate of soda can act as a protective barrier against urinary tract infections.

- **Fights gout and other joint problems:** By regulating blood pH and lowering uric acid levels, sodium bicarbonate water can be an effective remedy for gout and arthritis.
- **Increased physical performance:** Baking soda can help control the acidity produced during physical exercise, reducing muscle soreness and fatigue.
- **Control cholesterol levels:** Drinking sodium bicarbonate water could have a positive effect on reducing high levels of LDL cholesterol, known as 'bad cholesterol'.

It's important to mention that, despite these potential benefits, baking soda should be consumed with caution and moderation, due to its high sodium content, which may not be suitable for some people, particularly those with high blood pressure.

16. Massage ring

The acupressure ring is a self-massage accessory designed to relieve pain in the fingers. The ring is made up of triangles with rounded tips that stimulate the energy points on the fingers. Its use is directly inspired by the acupressure treatments of traditional Chinese medicine. This technique is based on the fact that the body is made up of thousands of points along energy channels known as meridians. Activating these points helps to rebalance the body's energies and relieve aches and pains, particularly if you are experiencing the following symptoms:

✖ Numbness
✖ Joint pain
✖ Regular cramps
✖ Fatigue
✖ Poor circulation

The acupressure ring is very easy to use. All you have to do is slide the ring over any finger and the pressure will be applied automatically thanks to the elastic band, which promotes compression. This compression is essential to activate your blood circulation, which will help your cells to regenerate. That's why, after a few moments, you'll feel warmth in your hand. This is a sign that the blood is circulating better in your fingers. Your hand will feel lighter and more relaxed. You'll also see your fingers gradually deflate. You can roll the ring along the entire length of your finger for self-massage. You only need to make ten passes over each finger to benefit from the ring's effects.

The hands are the parts of the body that are subject to the most strain. That's why when you're working on a computer, playing an instrument, doing the housework or gardening, the muscles in your hand are constantly contracting. The acupressure ring is also recommended for people who climb or do other activities that require them to work their grip. In fact, to have strength in your fingers for a good grip, your body's cells need to be well oxygenated. That means getting your blood flowing. What's more, by relieving pressure on the joints, the acupressure ring prevents arthritis problems.

The benefits of the massage ring

- ✔ Relieves fingers
- ✔ Promotes the well-being of the hands
- ✔ Activates blood circulation
- ✔ Fights numbness
- ✔ Alleviates joint pain
- ✔ Revitalising

Thanks to its elastic system, the acupressure ring fits any finger. It's made of stainless steel, so you can keep it on your finger without it getting damaged. To take full advantage of its soothing properties, the ring is made up of rounded triangles to exert pressure on the energy points on your finger without causing pain. What's more, it's easy to carry, so you can slip the acupressure ring around your finger at any time to benefit from its relaxing and analgesic virtues.

17. The benefits of yoga during Sec fasting cures

Dry fasting is a deeply purifying practice. To accompany and optimise this experience, yoga proves to be a precious ally. The combination of dry fasting and yoga can offer significant benefits for both body and mind.

- **Body-Mind Harmonisation Through Yoga During Dry Fasting**

During a dry fast, the body undergoes various changes and adaptations. Yoga, with its postures (asanas), breathing techniques (pranayama) and meditation, helps to maintain balance and strengthen the mind-body connection. It promotes relaxation, reduces stress and improves body awareness, which is particularly beneficial when fasting.

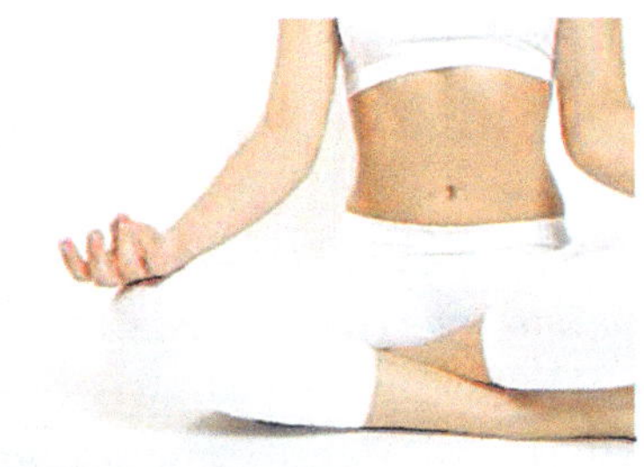

- ***Yoga postures adapted to dry fasting***

During a dry fast, certain yoga postures are particularly recommended for their gentleness and their ability to stimulate circulation, digestion and the elimination of toxins. Here are a few key postures:

1. **Tadasana (The Mountain):** This simple yet powerful posture helps to improve posture and balance, while

strengthening the legs and feet. It promotes body awareness and anchoring.

2. **Balasana (Child's Pose):** A relaxing posture that helps to calm the nervous system. It gently stretches the back, hips and thighs, which is beneficial during fasting.
3. **Viparita Karani (Legs against the Wall or Sarvangasana):** This gentle inversion promotes relaxation and blood circulation. It is ideal for relieving tired legs and improving digestion.
4. **Paschimottanasana (Sitting Pinch)**: This posture stretches the back of the body and helps to stimulate the digestive organs. It is beneficial for eliminating toxins and for relaxation.
5. **Supta Baddha Konasana (Reclining Goddess):** An open, relaxing posture for the hips and groin. It promotes deep relaxation and helps to release tension.

- ***Pranayama and Meditation During Dry Fasting***

In addition to asanas, pranayama (breathing techniques) and meditation play an important role during dry fasting. Pranayama helps to regulate vital energy (prana) and calm the mind, while meditation promotes concentration, mental clarity and inner peace.

- ***Integrate Yoga into your*** Dry ***Fasting Cure***

Incorporating yoga into your dry fasting cure can greatly enhance the experience. It is advisable to practise gentle yoga sessions adapted to your energy level during the fast. Listening to your body is essential to avoid overexertion. It is also important to hydrate properly before and after fasting.

In short, practising yoga during a dry fast offers multiple benefits, particularly in terms of relaxation, improving digestion and eliminating toxins, as well as strengthening the mind-body connection. Gentle postures and breathing and meditation practices are particularly well suited to accompanying and enriching the dry fasting experience.

18. Square breathing

Known as "Sama Vritti", square breathing is a breathing technique derived from pranayama (breath discipline) that helps you learn to control your breathing to reduce stress and improve your well-being. In less than five minutes, you can effectively calm yourself.

The virtues of square breathing are manifold. By voluntarily controlling our breathing, we can regulate our emotions and our well-being. Breathing has a powerful effect on the brain: square breathing improves blood oxygenation and the reflexes of the vegetative (involuntary) nervous system.

The Sama Vritti exercise also teaches you to better mobilise your respiratory muscles, particularly the diaphragm. Diaphragmatic breathing has many health benefits, particularly for mental health.

Square breathing is simple, natural and easy to do. It takes just a few minutes to feel its benefits and to improve physiological, physical and emotional balance. Like many breathing techniques, it is an effective way of relaxing while becoming aware of your body's respiratory needs. Remember, breathing is vital and plays an essential role in our well-being.

❤ The main benefits of Sama Vritti square breathing are:

- Reduces stress, anxiety and anguish (anti-stress and anxiolytic action);
- Helps you manage your emotions more effectively;
- Helps reduce depression;
- Improves blood oxygenation;
- Improves concentration;
- Promotes sleep;
- Relaxes the whole body (relaxation exercise);
- Raises awareness of the importance of breathing for health;
- Improves vegetative nervous system reflexes;

- Better mobilisation of the respiratory muscles and relaxation of the diaphragm;
- Gives you a bit of energy.

Square breathing is performed in four phases of equal duration: inhalation, retention (apnoea with full lungs), exhalation, retention (empty lungs). This combination should be performed several times, until you reach a state of inner calm, well-being and equanimity. Breathing is done through the nose only. Although a quiet place is ideal, any place is a good place to breathe consciously: at home, on public transport, at the gym, in a queue, with friends, at work... Don't miss out on this exercise with its fabulous benefits!

Anti-stress tip: imagine that with each inhalation you purify your body and with each exhalation you expel stress and all your problems. You can also aim for the prana that oxygenates the whole body.

The length of the four phases depends on your mood and how you feel. The four-second duration is often recommended because it suits the vast majority of people and ensures excellent results. Relaxation guaranteed! However, this figure can be adapted to suit your mood and increased as you progress. Bear in mind that ease is preferable to performance. Don't necessarily try to lengthen the phases. The square breathing exercise with well-executed four-second phases is very effective.

Example: four seconds inspiration + four seconds retention + four seconds exhalation + four seconds retention.

The number of repetitions also depends on how you feel. Generally speaking, it's advisable to do at least ten to feel the first real benefits. Twenty cycles is ideal. It's better to repeat the exercise two or three times a day, rather than doing too many repetitions at once, as this will be more effective. Square breathing is a simple exercise, accessible to everyone. All you have to do is relax and concentrate on your breathing.

19. Practising cardiac coherence

Breathe in through your nose for about five seconds as if your heart were inflating and then five seconds as if it were deflating. Your breathing should be purely abdominal. Do three times five minutes a day, or more if you feel like it. Put yourself in a spirit of joy when you do this. This breathing will calm the vagus nerve and reduce stress, heart rate and blood pressure. Be fully in the present when you do this.

The general effects are a regeneration of your energy, which helps to control emotions. A strengthening of the immune system induces a positive psychological state and an increase in immunoglobulin a. It also reduces general anxiety and harmonises vital biological functions such as digestive regulation and heart rate.

- **Visualisation: "I reconcile myself with my diseased organ", by Dr Rougier**
  - Lie down in a quiet place, or if that's not possible, sit comfortably or get into the coachman's position. Relax your body and close your eyes.
  - Take three deep breaths (always through your nose), then adopt a regular breathing rhythm, without forcing: inhale to the count of three (or one thousand, two thousand, three thousand...), then exhale slowly to the count of six (or one thousand, two thousand, three thousand...). Repeat three times.
  - Then imagine (visualise) your diseased organ. You have a choice when it comes to this representation: you can look up an image or photograph of the real organ in a dictionary or anatomy book and draw inspiration from it. You can also let your imagination run wild and create a more schematic or fanciful representation. The important thing is that the image 'speaks' to you.

- Next, send a wave of serenity towards the ailing organ. The image most commonly used for this purpose is that of a beautiful white (or golden) light, soothing and calming, bathing the diseased organ.
- Anchor this image by accompanying it with chosen words. Mentally repeat to the sick organ: "I am aware that you are suffering for me and I thank you for it. Then: "Now, I send you the strength of this light to help you recover." By saying these words, it's as if you're sending your body both gratitude and new healing forces (the two "mix" in the positive effects of psychosomatics).
- Repeat each phase of this visualisation seven times. Then concentrate again on your breathing rhythm until you return to normal consciousness and open your eyes.
- Warning: I'll say this often, but if you're not used to these therapeutic trainings, don't let your mind judge you, then immediately criticise you: "What you're doing is stupid", "It's a waste of time", "It's just words, childish things", "Words don't heal", etc. Bear in mind that everything great that has been achieved in this world has always been achieved through courage and "words". So, persevere serenely for at least ten days: that's the time you need to tame your over-critical thoughts stemming from your fearful (or pretentious!) subconscious.

20. Meditation session: Visualisation for physical and emotional healing

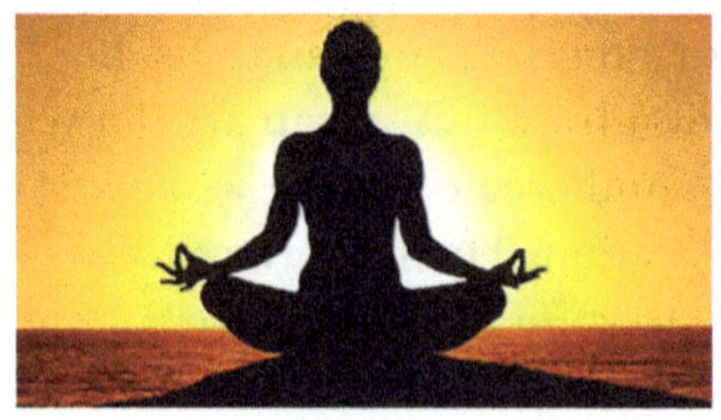

Sit down comfortably in a quiet place where you won't be disturbed. Close your eyes and take a few deep breaths, concentrating on the sensation of the air entering and leaving your lungs. Feel your body begin to relax. Now visualise a soft, soothing light descending from the sky and enveloping your whole being. This light represents healing and purity. Imagine this light penetrating every cell in your body, bringing health, vitality and well-being. Concentrate on the areas of your body that need healing. Visualise the light intensifying in these areas, repairing and revitalising every cell. Feel the pain, tension or illness dissipate, replaced by a feeling of comfort and strength.

Now turn your attention to your mind and emotions. Imagine that the light soothes your thoughts and brings clarity and serenity. Let go of any anxiety, sadness or anger, and visualise them dissolving in the light. Feel a sense of peace and balance settle over you. Stay in this state of relaxation and visualisation for as long as you like. When you are ready to end the session, take a few deep breaths and slowly return to awareness of your surroundings. Open your eyes, stretch gently and take a moment to appreciate the sense of renewal and healing you have created within yourself.

Feel free to tailor this session to your personal needs, focusing on the aspects of healing that are most relevant to you.

21. Chi Machine

The benefits of the Chi Machine massage therapy we use in our cures include temporary relief of minor muscle aches, pains and tension caused by fatigue or overwork. It temporarily stimulates circulation. It relaxes the muscles, which promotes a greater sense of well-being! According to an Australian study, it promotes lymphatic drainage and movement. Recent studies have even shown that massage can be beneficial against anxiety, stress, insomnia, fibromyalgia, lymphoedema and headaches. The current model is the SDM888 (replacing the SM330) which is also known as an aerobic exercise, passive aerobic exercise, Chi exercise or Chi exercise machine.

Dr Shizuo Inoue was President of the Japanese Association for Oxygen Health. With more than 38 years' experience, he developed and designed the Original Sun Ancon Chi machine. Dr Inoue's design was based on human physiology, allowing the body to work effortlessly with its natural frequencies. The machine's figure-eight goldfish movement allows maximum body movement without excessive pressure on the spine. The original Sun Ancon Chi machine has an oscillation speed of around 140 to 144 cycles per minute. This speed of oscillation is the speed that Dr Inoue found most beneficial for the circulatory system and for promoting general well-being. Dr Inoue expressed in his book *Aerobic Respiration Exercise and Health* that a lack of the body's ability to use oxygen properly could lead to pain, numbness, stiffness, itching and other signs of inflammation.

He also believed that if this state persisted in the body for long periods, it could lead to more serious health problems. Dr Jan Kirschner wrote: *"One of the wonderful benefits is that it allows the body to work effortlessly with its natural frequencies."* The 144 cycles per minute (oscillations) are both a multiple of the average heart rate (72) and brain speed, but also the rhythm of the spinal pump (12). Each person's body is influenced by all the physical, emotional, mental and chemical forces to which it is exposed, and by its ability to respond effectively to these forces. Because you are lying down, no tension is applied to any part of your body and there is no risk of injury. The machine is portable and easy to carry. It provides a maximum workout in a minimum amount of time. Dr Inoue's original Chi Machine design has been patented in several countries, including the USA (patent no. 510 7822), the UK, Japan, Germany and Australia. It is also registered as a medical device by Japanese Medical Affairs. In the United States, it is registered with the FDA as a therapeutic massage device. In Canada, it is registered as a Class II medical device. Health Canada believes that the benefits of the chi machine also include reducing fluid in the legs and extracellular fluid in the whole body, and providing a full body massage. A study carried out in

Australia is shared on Pubmed, showing how it has proved useful for people with chronic secondary lymphoedema of the legs.

The machine is useful if you do little physical exercise, have poor circulation, tired and aching muscles, general aches and pains, insomnia, menstrual pain or anaemia, or if you are overweight. It is also effective in cases of chronic inflammation, stress, poor digestion or constipation, bone spurs, nervousness, backache and lumbar pain, malfunctioning of the internal organs, asthma, and any chronic health problems.

22. The TESLA model 3D Schumann Plateau

The Schumann System does not produce harsh unnatural movements, unlike most traditional vibrating plates. It is a biodynamic energy system that mimics the natural fluidity of movement without the use of galvanic oz currents or chemicals. The system is based on the transmission of a gentle, three-dimensional sinusoidal oscillation amplitude rotating to the right and of a frequency to the whole body, in particular to the neuromuscular system.

- **Preventive and Beneficial**

The Schumann 3D System can rapidly help to reduce the pain caused by various disorders.

Here is a list of its virtues:

- Mental and physical well-being
- Action against mental and physical problems
- Prevent adhesions in connective tissue
- Increased stability of the spine and the entire bone system
- Improving the buffer function of intervertebral discs
- Activates lymphatic circulation and improves the immune system
- Greater joint freedom, improved mobility and elasticity

- Brings natural harmony to body and mind
- Activation of the metabolism (weight optimisation) and the entire supply of nutrients
- Relief from hip and shoulder pain
- Slimming the figure and improving the outward appearance of cellulite
- Activates and invigorates the skin by fine-tuning three-dimensional vibrations
- Regular use prevents the formation of new fatty deposits
- Improved quality of life and general well-being!
- Improved balance
- Prevention of falls and bills
- Reduced risk of cramps
- Increased ability to concentrate thanks to better blood supply to the brain and improved oxygenation
- Neutralisation of harmful environmental influences (electro-smog / stress)
- For restful, natural sleep and more energy during the day
- Safe running and optimum ground contact
- Improved reflexes
- Relaxing the nerves
- Removes blockages, increases energy flow
- The body regains its natural rhythm
- Promotes blood circulation
- Regulation of digestion
- Arthritis (inflammation of the joints)
- Herniated disc (disc prolapse)
- Burnout syndrome
- Cellulite
- Blood circulation disorders
- Relaxation problems
- Joint pain
- Lumbago
- Sciatica

- Headaches / Migraines (cephalalgia)
- Varicose veins
- Lumbar syndrome
- Incontinence
- Multiple sclerosis
- Lymphatic oedema
- Loss of libido
- Bekhterev's disease (ankylosing spondylitis)
- Neck contracture
- Nervousness
- Osteoporosis
- Parkinson (morbus Parkinson)
- Digestive problems
- Rheumatism
- Back pain
- Sleep disorders
- Stress
- Overweight
- Muscle tension

From a more energetic point of view

The 3D Schumann Plateau offers a treatment option by dissolving energy blockages. Whole-body oscillation stimulates energy points and meridians, bringing the energy system into balance. The aim of biodynamic massage on the Plateau Schumann 3D is to eliminate blockages and emotional contractions, so that physical well-being automatically follows. Sales and advice: www.jeunesec.com

- **For use throughout the year**

23. Fir balm: a treasure trove of health benefits

Baume de Sapin is a natural ally for healthy living. Made according to ancient traditions, it is a real concentrate of well-being. Cooked in a fir vat, this exceptional balm is a real gift from nature. Nicknamed "the doctor of the forest", it is a powerful ally for your health and youth.

- **Rich in Essential Nutrients**

Siberian fir needles, the balm's key ingredient, are loaded with ascorbic acid (320mg), tocopherol, tannins, phytoncides and resins. This unique blend helps to purify blood vessels, improving their elasticity and blood quality, while offering a detoxifying and remineralising effect.

- **A treasure trove of bio-active ingredients**

Baume de Sapin contains a multitude of essential organic active ingredients:

    - Vitamins: B, A, C, E
    - Minerals: calcium, iron, silicon, zinc, magnesium
    - Flavonoids, phytoncides, amino acids, organic acids, sterols, chlorophyll, cellulose, anthocyanins, coumarins, borneol, safrole, tannin compounds, polysaccharides, polyprenols

- **Prevention and cure: a winning combination**

Fir extract is renowned for its exceptional preventive properties. This biologically active substance promotes healing, strengthens the immune system and increases the body's resistance to disease.

- **Exquisite taste and therapeutic properties**

Fir resin, with its remarkable taste properties, adds a unique flavour to drinks and desserts. Young fir shoots, carefully extracted in ecologically pure regions, enrich the balm with a host of active substances.

- **Antiseptic and anti-inflammatory properties**

Fir Balm stimulates the elimination of necrotic tissue and toxins, speeding up cell regeneration and wound healing. It also activates the excretory and lymphatic systems, purifying the body and normalising metabolic processes.

- **Why use Baume de Sapin?**

Ideal as a diluted drink, Baume de Sapin:

- Speeds healing of gastric ulcers and gastritis
- Eliminates vitamin deficiencies
- Increases the body's resistance
- Freshens breath and prevents dental problems

External use for various ailments

Applied as an ointment, Fir Balm helps to treat:

- Burns, irritations, eczema
- Purulent wounds, fungal infections

Recommended dosage

- Prevention: 1 teaspoon 1 to 2 times a day
- Treatment: 1 tablespoon per 1 litre of water, 3 times a day.
- Colds, flu: 1 teaspoon + 1-5 drops in 100mg of water, 3 times a day.
- Oncology: 5 tablespoons a day

Antiseptic and anti-inflammatory properties: Siberian fir resin has strong antiseptic and anti-inflammatory properties, making it effective in preventing and treating bacterial and viral infections. It is often used to treat wounds, cuts, burns and skin irritations.

1. **Effect on the respiratory system:** Resin is good for the respiratory system. It can help relieve the symptoms of colds, flu, bronchitis and other respiratory disorders. It is also used to clear the airways and make breathing easier.

2. **Immune system boost**: Resin components such as phytoncides can help boost the immune system, making it more resistant to infection and disease.
3. **Antioxidant properties**: Fir resin contains natural antioxidants that help fight free radicals in the body, reducing oxidative stress and preventing premature ageing and certain chronic diseases.
4. **Pain relief:** Thanks to its analgesic properties, fir resin can help relieve pain, particularly joint and muscle pain and headaches.
5. **Improved Skin Health:** Resin is beneficial for the skin, helping to treat various skin conditions such as eczema, psoriasis and dermatitis. It also promotes wound healing and contributes to healthy, radiant skin.
6. **Relaxing and calming effects:** The aroma of Siberian fir resin can have a calming and relaxing effect, helping to reduce stress and anxiety.
7. **Expectorant properties:** It is often used in the treatment of respiratory ailments due to its expectorant properties, which help expel mucus and secretions from the respiratory tract.

Product available at www.jeunesec.com
https://www.jeunesec.com/boutique-en-ligne.html?store-page=R%C3%A9sine-de-sapin-de-sib%C3%A9rie-Lot-de-3-pots-p553446113

24. Neem

Neem, known scientifically as Azadirachta indica, is a tree native to India, where it has been used for thousands of years in Ayurvedic medicine for its medicinal properties. Neem powder is obtained by grinding the dried leaves of this tree.

- **Properties and active ingredients**

Neem powder is rich in bioactive compounds, including limonoids, triterpenes, antioxidants and nitrogen compounds, which are responsible for its medicinal properties. Among these compounds, azadirachtin is particularly well known for its insecticidal and anti-parasitic action.

- **Benefits**

1. **Antibacterial and antifungal effect**: Neem powder is renowned for its antibacterial and antifungal properties. It helps to combat various skin infections such as acne, fungal infections and boils.
2. **Skin care:** Rich in vitamins and antioxidants, it nourishes the skin, reduces the signs of ageing and improves radiance.
3. **Treatment of dental problems:** Used in powder form or as a mouthwash, its antibacterial properties help combat plaque, cavities and gum disease.
4. **Anti-parasite action**: Effective against internal and external parasites, including intestinal worms and lice.
5. **Relief from skin conditions**: Used to treat eczema, psoriasis and other inflammatory skin conditions.
6. **Diabetes control:** Neem powder can help regulate blood glucose levels, making it useful in the management of diabetes.
7. **Boosts the immune system:** Its immunostimulant properties help to strengthen the body's natural defences.

- **Dosage and precautions**

Neem powder can be used in a variety of ways, including topical application to the skin, infusion, or ingestion in capsule form. The dosage depends on the use and the form in which it is consumed. It is advisable to follow the recommendations of a health professional for safe and effective use, adapted to each individual situation. Although neem is generally safe for most adults when used appropriately, it can cause certain side effects such as allergic reactions. It is not recommended for pregnant and breast-feeding women.

25 Photo Light Therapy (Ecolight device) and its benefits during Therapeutic Dry Fasting and for day-to-day treatment

Introduction

Our therapeutic dry fasting centre is a pioneer in the use of the Ecolight light therapy device. This technology, invented in the 1980s by Dr Y.M. Belyaev, is distinguished by its use of ultraviolet light (305-405 nm) in pulsed mode. This innovation offers significant immunostimulant, bactericidal, vitamin-enhancing, healing and anti-inflammatory effects.

History and scientific recognition

The Ecosve device has received the approval of several eminent Russian scientists. These include Academician V.I. Shumakov of the Russian Academy of Sciences, Corresponding Member S.V. Gautier, and Academician A.N. Razumov, who validated the methodological recommendations. The project's scientific director was A.T. Bykov, corresponding member of the Russian Academy of Medical Sciences and Major General of the Medical Service.

Development and production

After more than 20 years of research, it was not until 2008 that the Ecosve technology began to be mass-produced in Russia. Prior to this crucial step, rigorous testing of the medical light therapy device was carried out in various medical establishments, including the FGU "VNII tests of medical equipment" Rosdravnazor RF, the FGU "NIIT and IO Rosmedtechnologii", and the FGU "Central Clinical Sanatorium named after F.E.

Dzerzhinsky". Trials also took place in six departments of the Kuban State Medical University.

Expansion and use

The Ecolight device is currently operating successfully in over 100 medical institutions and sanatoria across Russia, including Moscow, the Moscow region, Krasnodar, the Krasnodar and Stavropol territories, Rostov-on-Don and Chelyabinsk.

Biomolecular mechanisms of action of UV blood irradiation (UVOC)

UVOC (ultraviolet blood irradiation) is a method of influencing the blood using quanta of ultraviolet light, which has been used in medicine for more than 80 years. In 1928, V. Hancock and E. Knott performed the first extracorporeal UVOC sessions on a pregnant woman suffering from septicaemia. In the USSR, this method was applied for the first time in 1937 in Leningrad by transfusologists Filatov A.N. and Kasumov G.I. Later, in 1979, the Leningrad State Optical Institute developed and tested the "Izolda" MD-73 device, which is still in use today.

The mechanism of action of UV irradiation of blood is complex and varied. UV light enables the molecules in the cells of living organisms to absorb quanta of radiation, thereby participating in photochemical reactions that modify their structure and functions. UV irradiation of blood increases its bactericidal activity, inactivates toxic substances and enzymes, and activates blood cell functions. These combined effects improve microcirculation and increase the oxygenation capacity of the blood.

Therapeutic effects of UVOC

UVOC has several therapeutic effects:

- Bactericide: UV rays have a bactericidal effect on the blood, similar to that of antibiotics.
- Anti-inflammatory: UVOC reduces inflammation and stimulates immune defence processes.

- Improved microcirculation: Blood viscosity is reduced, improving blood circulation.
- Increased oxygenation capacity: Irradiated blood transports oxygen better to organs and tissues.
- Stimulation of regenerative and metabolic processes: UVOC promotes cell regeneration and normalises metabolic processes.
- Immunocorrective: UVOC restructures the immune system, improving non-specific immune responses.
- Stimulation of erythrocyte regeneration: Improves the functional properties of red blood cells.

Indications for use of the Ecolight device
The Ecolight device is recommended for a variety of medical conditions, including:

- Allergic diseases
- Atherosclerosis
- Viral herpes
- Purulent-inflammatory diseases
- Hypertension
- Endarteritis obliterans
- Type 2 diabetes
- Muscle injuries, sprains, haematomas
- Gastritis and peptic ulcer disease
- Bronchitis and pleurisy
- Pancreatitis and cholecystitis
- Gout
- Post-operative debility
- Injuries, fractures, burns
- Acne
- Neurodermatitis and dermatitis
- Psoriasis
- Rheumatoid arthritis
- Dry eye syndrome
- Ischaemic heart disease

- Chronic fatigue syndrome
- Decreased libido and impotence
- Varicose veins
- Prevention of acute respiratory illnesses and influenza

Clinical results and application methods

Clinical studies on polychromatic light pulse therapy (PSIT) began in 1985. Dr Y.M. Belyaev, who designed the method and the device, carried out this research in collaboration with several clinics in Krasnodar and other cities such as Sochi, Anapa and Moscow. The results showed that PSIT is effective in modulating and correcting immunity, increasing the body's protective properties and restoring its lost immune status.

Observed and validated clinical effects

- Inflammatory diseases: Increase in the body's anti-inflammatory potential and stimulation of immune defence processes.
- Allergic diseases: Correction of immune status with a lasting anti-allergenic effect lasting from several months to three to four years.
- Psoriasis, Eczema, Seborrhoea: Normalises immunological processes and cleanses the affected skin.
- Ischaemic heart disease: Reduces atherogenic lipid indicators, improves blood supply and oxygenation, lowers blood pressure and improves metabolism.
- Rheumatoid arthritis: Reduction in the biological activity of the disease, improvement in psycho-emotional state, reduction in pain syndrome, and increased functional capacity of the joints.
- Viral herpes: Rapid disappearance of symptoms such as itching and burning, reduction in the duration of the pain syndrome and prolongation of the inter-relational period.

- Eye diseases: Therapeutic effect due to its anti-inflammatory and trophostimulant action, improving the state of microcirculation in the lacrimal organs.
- Chronic fatigue: effect on energy and mitochondria and improvement of sporting performance.
- Circulation: improves capillaries and circulation in general.
- Immunity: general immunomodulating effect

Contraindications

Use of the Ecolight device is contraindicated in cases of hypersensitivity to UVB, porphyria, thrombocytopenia, hypocoagulation, acute cerebral circulatory disorders, very serious liver and kidney diseases, hyperthyroidism, lupus erythematosus.

General information

This therapy can be used on a daily basis to maintain health, for prevention and of course before, during or after dry fasting for consolidation. It is of course optional during fasting but can be discussed with the person accompanying the dry fast, but it can be of significant interest during cures for oxygenation, general tone and inflammation. Circulatory improvement during dry fasting and general homeostasis.

Shop sales and instructions for use: Ecolight device www,jeunesec

CHAPTER 18

Transformation and healing through group dry fasting

In today's Western world, where stress and lifestyle-related illness are omnipresent, traditional methods of healing and well-being are gaining in popularity. Among these practices, holistic dry fasting, practised in groups in specialised centres around the world, offers a unique transformational experience. This chapter explores the emotional and physical transformations experienced through interpersonal relationships for individuals who participate in these dry fasting cures, focusing on the profound impact of the group effect in the self-healing process.

This method is not based solely on dry fasting therapy derived from Russian methods. In Western countries, we base our lifestyles on a very mental view of the world. It is therefore necessary to go through the mental pathway in order to become aware of the cause of our illnesses, and communication is a decisive factor in this. Dry fasting encourages a very powerful process of introspection that brings out messages from the unconscious, which are often revealed through group sharing.

This is why, from the moment they arrive at the retreat, fasters are enveloped in a cocoon of kindness and security. This is the basis and foundation of any openness to the introspection necessary for self-healing. In this space, where everything is designed for comfort and tranquillity, there's nothing to manage, just to relax and focus on your own well-being. This feeling of security is crucial: it allows the fasting person to let go of everyday concerns and immerse themselves fully in their inner healing process. Getting out of the box is a vital part of relaxing the mind and allowing the waters of the body – our emotions – to be released.

1. Safety and Focus

Physically, dry fasting acts as a centrifugal force, from the inside out, mobilising and eliminating the miasmas, toxic and energetic waste that are deeply rooted in the body and operating afterwards as a unique system of self-healing and self-repair of the body via the stem cells. But dry fasting also works on a much more subtle level, helping to free the body's water of its emotional memories accumulated over the years, as well as trans-generational memories. Each dry fasting retreat undertaken enables a deeper cleansing, like peeling layers of onions. The safe environment of the centre and the guides help the fasters to concentrate solely on these internal processes of elimination and self-repair, without any external distractions.

The group effect is a healing force in itself on several levels that we try to bring to the fore. I've seen too many groups in Russia and elsewhere that were completely broken up, where there were no workshops for sharing, where the fasters were just a number and their feelings could never really be released. One of the most powerful aspects of dry fasting for me is the energising group effect. Far from feeling isolated, the dry fasters are constantly surrounded by people who share their journey and their difficulties during the transformative process, and mirror effects come into play in the stories of the participants which resonate with their personal journey. This solidarity and need to belong is nurtured during the practice and creates a group dynamic that is not only reassuring, but also intensely healing.

Participants support and encourage each other, sharing their experiences and trials. This support is all the more important as dry fasting can be both an initiatory and transformative experience. The group effect ensures that individual fasters never feel alone and that morale remains high, facilitating an environment where everyone can gain maximum benefit.

Our therapeutic dry fasting retreats are a unique model and offer a wide range of therapies and workshops to facilitate the practice of dry fasting, while being conscious of creating an exchange with other participants between giving and receiving. These proven methods are integrated to maximise organ renewal and toxin elimination. These biotherapies have evolved and adapted over the years, with new methods being added to and improved.

2. Therapies and Workshops

- **Biotherapy and Care Systems:** On-site treatments such as bio-resonance, ito-thermia, Schumann trays, therapeutic blankets and chi machines speed up the healing process.
- **Personal development:** Conscious walking workshops, personal development circles, yoga sessions and individual emotional release sessions are designed to help fasters let go of their emotions and regenerate more effectively. Gentle massage restores the body's energy, while massages that are too strong take energy away from the body. The therapist will find the right balance on an individual basis.

These activities are essential for obtaining results that are approximately 40 to 60% better than those of a solo fast, according to the testimonies of fasters who have experimented in their own homes or with us. The group creates an environment where the faster can relax completely and where the alchemy of healing operates on both physical and subtle levels.

The process of dry fasting in a group is comparable to the transformation of the phoenix: the fasting person rises from the ashes at the end of the cure. Throughout this period, group activities help to speed up the passage of time, while giving priority to total rest. This is because our two energy guzzlers – the body and the mind – are put on pause.

Thanks to this internal alchemy, the fasting person is freed from the burdens of the past and regenerated in a profound way. The support team plays a key role in providing constant care and security, allowing fasters to let themselves be lulled into this transformation.

The group dry fasting cure we offer is more than just a physical detoxification method. It is a holistic experience that transforms the individual on every level: physical, emotional, mental and spiritual. Thanks to the group effect and the many therapeutic supports, every faster goes through this experience not only successfully, but also with a profound inner transformation. In the end, everyone emerges not only healthier, but also more in tune with themselves and ready to continue their journey with a new perspective. This method should be disseminated everywhere as a unique system of physical and psychic healing that our humanity so badly needs.

3. From Mind to Heart, unfolding your authenticity

As we said earlier, the dry faster finds themselves in a very powerful centrifugal force which leads them to extract themselves from their mind and rest their body. With the mind no longer having the energy it needs to concentrate, an inner dynamic emerges and manifests itself, namely the intelligence of the heart, which reveals itself by opening the door to our emotions. It's impossible not to be overwhelmed by this emotional flow, which is usually controlled by the mind, and which frees itself. And it is through the group that each of us authentically expresses what we feel, as well as our personal history.

These talking circles are therapy in themselves. Because each person, echoing the other, will act in a perfect systemic way to help him or her untie their own wounds. No longer subject to the fear of the other, they can assert themselves with authenticity in their own truth. Without judgement, participants feel free to be themselves, and the barriers and limitations of the mind fall away, returning us to who we are: listening, caring beings.

Listening is a quality intrinsic to the success of these group workshops. No longer dependent on what the other person thinks, no longer obliged to justify themselves, but in a supportive and reassuring environment, each participant takes the time to listen to the other, despite their tiredness, and everyone emerges a better person for it. After all, how long has it been since we've had the opportunity to pay sincere attention to what we're going through, to what ails us and to our past? A group with its heart wide open allows everyone to be welcomed in all their parts, both beautiful and painful.

4. Frame and Contemplation

There's nothing better for starting a dry fast than to find yourself in an unusual environment in the midst of a caring group. That's why we offer several locations around the world with different characteristics, so that everyone can combine a holiday with a rejuvenating retreat.

Contemplation is an essential part of letting go of the mind and returning to the space of the heart. When we step out of our daily routines, in an unfamiliar place, with people we don't know, we are led to open our minds and our hearts. This process is like stepping out of our comfort zone, which makes it easier to open up to the world. It's through this first step that each of us, to the best of our knowledge and belief, can make a success of our fasting. That's why fasting at home is much less powerful than fasting in a group, outside the usual environment and in a lovely, safe setting.

The Benefits of Energy Healing During Dry Fasting: Advantages and Mechanisms

What is Energy Healing?

Energy healing is an ancient and holistic practice aimed at harmonizing the vital energy that surrounds and flows through our bodies. By using this energy, the practitioner, often called an energy healer, seeks to rebalance and smooth the energy flows within the client's body. This method, known since antiquity, can have profound effects on physical pain, emotions, and mental states through interaction with the etheric energy body.

Mechanisms of Energy Healing

The therapist interacts with the client's etheric energy body, a subtle dimension reflecting overall health. By focusing on this energy layer, the practitioner can detect and correct imbalances. The practitioner's hands pass over the client's body, without touching, to capture and redistribute energy in a balanced way. This process can:

1. **Reduce physical pain**: By releasing energy disturbances, energy healing can reduce muscle tension and chronic pain.
2. **Balance emotions**: Repressed emotions or traumas can be stored in the body. By restoring energy harmony, these

emotions can be released, bringing a sense of peace and clarity.

3. **Improve mental states**: The conventions and mental imagery used by the practitioner can induce deep relaxation states, reducing stress and anxiety.

Benefits of Energy Healing

Energy healing offers numerous benefits that touch various aspects of our being:

- **Emotional**: Stress relief, reduced anxiety, improved emotional stability.
- **Physical**: Reduced muscle tension, improved digestive issues, aid with sleep disorders.
- **Intellectual**: Clearer thoughts, improved concentration and creativity.
- **Spiritual**: Chakra realignment, purification of negative energies, enhanced spiritual connection.

Enhancing Dry Fasting Retreats

During dry fasting retreats, energy healing can be applied to enhance the effects of fasting. This combination allows for both physical and psychological releases, facilitating deeper detoxification and energy regeneration. Dry fasting, by its intense nature, can be supported by these treatments to improve energy flow, reduce fasting side effects, and help maintain optimal energy balance. Additionally, energy healing restores energy during dry fasting and calms the nervous system, providing extra support during this demanding period. During our dry fasting retreats, we offer these treatments for those who wish to receive them.

The Role and Stance of the Therapist

The therapist adopts a humble posture, not seeking to heal the client but to promote, through their knowledge, the proper flow of energy. This respectful and non-intrusive approach helps the client regain their natural balance and activate their own self-healing abilities. By facilitating energy harmonization, the practitioner acts as a guide and support, allowing vital energy to flow freely and effectively within the client's body.

The Course of an Energy Healing Session

An energy healing session begins with a preliminary interview where the practitioner and the client discuss the reasons for the consultation and the client's expectations. This dialogue helps to tailor the treatment personally.

The practitioner then proceeds by passing their hands along the client's body, detecting energy imbalances. Areas lacking energy are revitalized, while areas with excess energy are calmed. At the end of the session, an exchange takes place to discuss feelings and immediate effects.

Magnetism Session

Magnetism is a complementary practice to energy healing. Using magnetic passes, hand imposition, and breath, the magnetizer works to rebalance the client's energy bodies, glands, and organs. The magnetizer detects and regulates blockages, restoring the organs' ability to regulate and self-heal.

Precautions and Complementarity

It is important to note that energy healing and magnetism do not replace allopathic medicine. An energy healer or magnetizer will not make medical diagnoses or ask to interrupt ongoing treatment. However, these practices can be effective complements, providing additional support for healing and general well-being.

Conclusion

Energy healing and magnetism offer a holistic approach to harmonizing the body, mind, and soul. By smoothing energy and eliminating disturbances, they bring relaxation, inner peace, and vitality. Experience these treatments for purification of the being, chakra balancing, and the release of negative energies. Say goodbye to stress and emotional blockages with this ancient and powerful practice.

By integrating energy healing into your wellness routine, and especially during dry fasting retreats, you open the door to better self-understanding and a more harmonious balance of your vital energy.

CHAPTER 19

Emerging from dry fasting

1. Possible complications after dry fasting

It is essential to fully understand and manage the potential complications when resuming eating after dry fasting, especially if it is of long duration. Here is an improved and reorganised presentation of possible complications and their solutions:

1. **Overeating and controlling food cravings.** After a dry fast, it is crucial to avoid overeating. Overeating can be catastrophic and is often unconscious. In a controlled setting where the first meals are provided, this problem is better managed. In the event of excess, it is advisable to induce vomiting, use mild laxatives or natural remedies to cleanse the stomach.
2. **Post-fasting diet.** Start with one soup, then gradually increase to two soups a day, spacing meals out by at least six hours (for example, at 12pm and 6pm). Avoid foods that are too heavy, carbohydrates that are not chewed, and inappropriate preparations. Consider foods low in FODMAPs and avoid excess raw foods.
3. **Oedema and urine retention.** These problems occur when the body, having expended potassium during the fast, reacts negatively to the intake of salty foods at the start of the recovery. To remedy this, avoid salty foods, fast with water, use remedies such as Silicea med or laxative plants,

and consider a sauna after 24 hours to eliminate excess sodium.

4. **Minerals and proteins**. It is important to include minerals such as fir resin, magnesium and spirulina, as well as bio-available proteins, to help the body recover.
5. **Constipation**. If you are unable to defecate naturally for more than three to five days, consider an enema or the use of natural remedies such as Pianto or aloe vera. Physical activity such as walking or yoga, as well as laxative plants, can also help.
6. **Gas and digestive disorders:** To avoid these inconveniences, limit your carbohydrate intake after fasting, combine foods correctly and eat a suitable diet.

Finally, it is crucial to progress gradually in the practice of dry fasting, to study the resources available, to share experiences, and above all to monitor yourself carefully. Seek advice from someone with experience in this field and communicate with your companion about your activities during the fast. If symptoms of illness worsen during fasting, it may be advisable to continue fasting until they disappear, or to take specific measures when you resume eating if it is impossible to continue fasting.

2. When you come out of dry fasting, follow these important rules

As we mentioned at the outset, the correct way of exiting the fast is no less important than the fast itself. What's more, an incorrect exit can cancel out the beneficial effects of the fast you've already done. In other words, if you overeat when you come off the fast, all your ills will return. In fact, if you overeat on leaving the fast and eat the wrong foods, you fill your body's cells with food debris that you won't be able to assimilate.

So beware of overeating when you come out of the fast, remember that coming out of the fast is in fact the second part.

If you eat too much after the fast, it is better not to start the fast. The correct exit from the fast represents 70% of the effectiveness of dry fasting.

One day of dry fasting is equivalent to three to five days of wet fasting. So, if you do a ten-day fast, you should ideally be out of the fast for two months. Throughout this period, it's best not to eat anything too heavy and to avoid indigestible, industrial and sugary foods. The body will continue to be cleansed and the cellular reset will be optimal.

Firstly, you need to drink water at a temperature of between 37 and 50 degrees, ideally. This water should come from a spring and be lukewarm all day long. It's also important to know how to drink. On the first day, you can add a natural probiotic such as Regulat, which we have on site. Half a teaspoon in water for two days or more. It will work on the intestinal microflora. And the vital thing is to drink slowly, sip by sip, and so on for eight hours. You need to drink according to your abilities. Some people will drink less, others more. If nausea or discomfort in the gastrointestinal tract is bothering you, you can take a little Sorbent such as Gel Silicea med, one tablespoon in water. It's easy to find in chemists. The best thing to do is to take diluted Pianto, but wait at least two or three days after coming off dry fasting as it's a bit salty. You can then brush your teeth. Drinking water can be combined with a hot shower or bath. As well as washing your teeth, you should continue to drink water during the day, followed by herbal teas.

In the afternoon, you can drink herbal teas such as nettle to drain the kidneys and gently add minerals. Then, perhaps take a teaspoon of good-quality spirulina in a shaker, if you know how it's made. Fir resin is used as a basifying agent and also provides minerals. In the evening or at lunchtime the next day, you can have a vegetable soup with ground courgette or two simple vegetables. You can also continue hydrating for one or two weeks, depending on your energy and weight reserves, but you need to be sure that you're getting back to eating properly and that your workload isn't too heavy.

After the soups come the cooked vegetables. Watch what happens. The key is to chew well. Put the fork down after each bite or use Chinese chopsticks. If you want to cut ketosis, you can eat Konjac, quail eggs, fish or perhaps a little buckwheat.

You can add salt to your food from the fourth day of fasting. It's best to use rock or sea salt, very gradually, the ideal dose being the tip of a knife.

Food should be varied and rich in vitamins, micro- and macro-elements. For the first five days following the start of the dry fast, use only fresh, clean, organic and high-quality produce. Do not consume sugar, products containing sugar or canned goods. The idea is to continue in ketosis, so if you can still manage a week without carbohydrates, that's ideal.

From the second day onwards, you can take a teaspoon of fir resin, which will provide minerals, alkalise and continue the cellular drainage process, while at the same time blocking the intestinal barrier. Be careful about the dose at the start, don't take too much as the resin is concentrated and bitter. This bitter taste will prevent you from craving sweet foods and delay the intake of these foods as long as possible. Raw foods can be eaten after three days of recovery. Many fasting centres offer raw food resumption, the worst being fruit, which is not suitable for a proper recovery. What's more, they will quickly stimulate your sweet cravings and raise your insulin levels, with all the problems that entails. There will also be too many abrasive fibres on the mucous membranes. After a week of dry fasting, the body will have to reheat its food, which will take up a lot of your energy, which will not be redistributed to the body to continue the detox and renew tissues and organs to their maximum. Fruit and salads can therefore be eaten after three days, but this will immediately stop the secretion of ketone bodies, so it's up to you. If you're really hungry in the morning, have an apple at 9am or some raw or cooked vegetables, then eat your meal at 12pm. Be prepared for the fact that your fingers and toes will be a little cold when you leave. Above all, stop taking cold or affusion baths. If the sea is warm, you can bathe without any problem. Your eyesight may also deteriorate, but it will return to normal as a result of the intense cleansing that has just taken place. People who normally have dry skin will find that their skin becomes even drier during fasting. The skin on the face and nose may crack during dry fasting, but hydration will return afterwards. You can apply various castor oil masks, which will significantly improve the skin.

At the end of the dry fast, you can carry out honey massages, which we explain below, to accelerate the cleansing of the body and improve lymphatic drainage. The biotherapies practised during our cures will help to prevent the blood from thickening and to restart the work of the organs which will have shrunk during the dry fast. The Schumann plateau, chi machine, yoga, walking and therapeutic blanket are also recommended.

When you emerge from dry fasting, particularly in the first few days, the immune system is rebuilt. The body is weakened at first, but then it will be rebuilt and immunity will become even stronger than before the dry fast.

It is a mistake to assume that a single dry fast, even a long-term one of around ten days, can completely cleanse the body of all toxins and thus regenerate the whole organism, curing a chronic pathology that has existed for years. Generally speaking, if you are highly intoxicated, two courses of treatment over six months is the minimum. Toxins that have accumulated over the years cannot be eliminated immediately, but only over a period of several days or weeks. It is important to understand that the more toxins you have removed before the dry fasting cure, the easier and more comfortable the fast will be. In chronic illnesses, three cures over a period of one year are necessary to achieve a tangible improvement. But if you're in good shape and free of disease, one cure a year will be enough to ensure good prevention.

Everything depends on persistence in achieving a stable therapeutic effect. A prerequisite for this persistence is the annual repetition of the preventive fasting cycle and, if necessary, the performance of a series of (fractional) fasts over several years in succession to achieve the final cure. There are many striking examples of how apparently doomed patients, stubbornly continuing to repeat long fasting treatments, became healthy people within a few years.

3. Feeding programme following long dry fasting

After dry fasting, you can quickly and easily re-establish proper digestion. Stick to the following rule: don't eat after 7pm. Avoid the starch-protein combination, which is the most complicated, especially during the first two weeks and ideally for as long as possible.

You can also choose to continue in ketosis by reducing all forms of carbohydrate as much as possible, including fruit, as this will prolong the effect of the fast. Avoid all sweet products. Choose Konjac as a plant to maintain the ketosis mechanism. You can eat all vegetables except potatoes and carrots. In this way, the body's self-cleansing process will take place and body fat will be normalised. Consider chicken stock if you have the time and patience. Put a whole organic chicken in a large saucepan and boil for two hours. Then put a three-quarters-full bottle in the fridge or freezer and eat the chicken. This is the basis of the GAPS diet, which aims to correct any dysbiosis. The broth helps to heal the mucous membranes by providing glutamine, an essential amino acid for the digestive barrier. It is also found in carob powder.

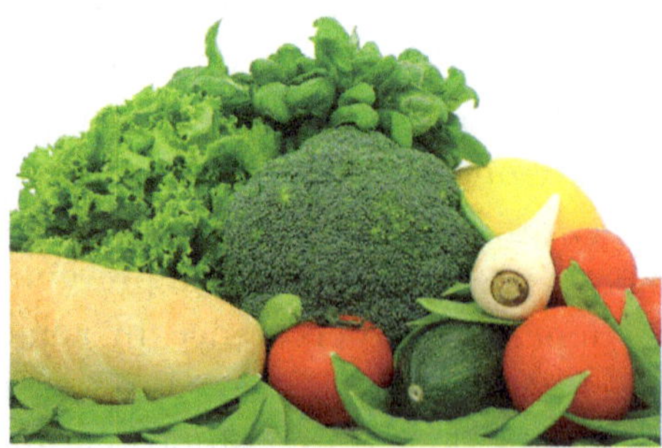

Do intermittent fasting and eat only at midday, as I have been doing for a long time. Always start with vegetable soup as your first meal, followed by larger cooked vegetables for two days. The types of vegetable suggested are those on the fodmaps list, i.e. the least fermentable. Then eat a fresh vegetable salad from Day 3, or steamed vegetables in winter. Carrots and green vegetables are a good stimulant for the digestive tract, as they cultivate the appropriate microflora and, through feedback, restore the endocrine system. Eat the salad and cooked vegetables together first. This will help to activate a number of processes that underpin the body's normal functioning. Don't forget to drink as much as you can during the day – prepare solar water, magnetised water, hand-informed water or Koltosov plates.

Observe the difference between raw, steamed and blanched for five minutes, whichever you tolerate better, your body will feel it straight away. Raw food stimulates the secretion of digestive juices but can be irritating for some people, as raw vegetables are rich in natural stimulants. You will feel that your body prefers this or that food. In winter, steaming will be a priority. As a result, you can increase your consumption of fresh vegetables to 80% of your diet, as they are very rich in vitality. Their tissues support the structure of body tissue and the elasticity of the skin.

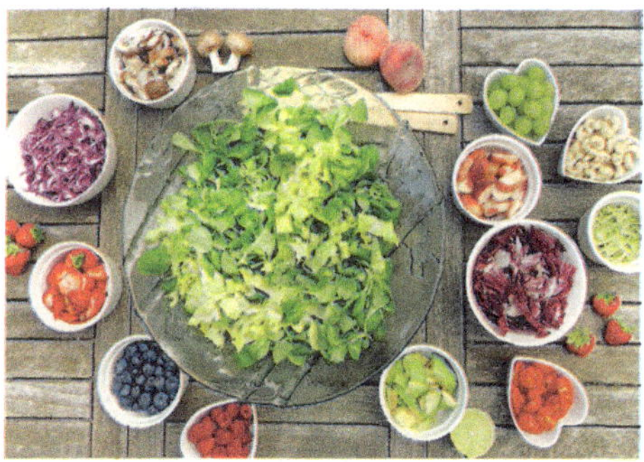

The ideal diet consists of 50% raw and cooked vegetables. Cellulose and pectin, contained in the majority of plant products, are called ballast substances because they are not absorbed by the body. These substances are necessary because they play an important role in the digestion process and in retaining water in the colon: they set up the intestinal hormonal system and through it the whole body, by regulating the motor function of the intestine. They create a favourable microflora in the gastrointestinal tract. Twenty per cent of your diet should come from protein foods, with preference given to fish. Protein can be in the form of fish, eggs or quail. Avoid coffee and industrial products for two months, and avoid gluten and dairy products as much as possible.

People who are prone to obesity should avoid eating fast or even slow sugars in the evening, or consume them in minimal quantities. A person absorbs three to five times more cereals than necessary. This leads to obesity. If you consume a small quantity, chewing it until it resembles milk, constipation disappears, intestinal peristalsis improves (when chewing, peristalsis is accelerated four times) and congestion in the digestive tract is eliminated.

It should be remembered that the recovery processes in the body after dry fasting continues for around one to three months, depending on the duration of the dry fast, and throughout this time the body must be given food of the highest possible quality to replenish itself.

It's best to exclude red meat and dairy products from your diet for as long as possible. From Day 3 onwards, eat fish and eggs. This will allow the body to continue its own protein biosynthesis for a while and increase the effect after fasting. Gradually, during the second and third weeks out, the number of meals should be normalised to three a day, trying to take care of its quality, but two meals are more than enough. Ideally, separate proteins from carbohydrates at each meal. In short, have one meal with quinoa and cooked vegetables, for example, and another meal with fish and cooked vegetables.

It is strictly forbidden to eat too much. Chew 20 times and use chopsticks if you want to slow down easily. Overeating can cause nausea and vomiting. The body is overloaded with food to which it is not yet accustomed, which causes this type of side effect.

The amount of salt should be increased gradually and it is preferable to use fleur de sel. An overdose taken at the end of a dry fast can cause swelling of the legs and arms and bags under the eyes. In addition, urine output falls sharply, frequent headaches occur and weight increases (by around 2kg during the day).

Foods rich in carbohydrates, particularly pure sugars, should be excluded. There is an acute spasm of the capillaries which, on impact with carbohydrates, causes dizziness, nausea, weakness, fatigue and also a feeling of drunkenness. Similarly, be sure to exclude all canned foods.

To cleanse the body thoroughly, it is necessary to take mixed turpentine baths according to Zalmanov when coming out of fasting. The total number of baths is ten, with one bath every three days. This bath comes from Russia with a much higher dosage than what you'll find on the French market, so I don't have a brand to recommend.

4. The benefits of food combinations after fasting

The following list presents the dissociated diet, based on the principles of Dr Shelton, who suggests not mixing certain types of food to optimise digestion and assimilation of nutrients, minimise digestive problems and improve general health.

Key points and objectives of the dissociated diet:

- Do not combine certain foods.
- Favour foods that are digested in a similar way in the same meal.
- Objectives: better digestion, more energy, prevention of fermentation and certain diseases.

Principles of the dissociated system:

- Do not mix acidic foods (proteins) with alkaline starchy foods.
- Specific digestion time for each food category.
- Eat the fruit on its own and some of it should not be mixed together.
- Vegetables and starchy foods can be combined.

- Limited consumption of dairy products.

Recommended food combinations:

- Animal proteins and vegetables (no starchy foods).
- Starches and vegetables (no protein).
- Fruit only.

Advantages of the dissociated diet:

- No foods excluded, no quantity limit.
- Simplified meal preparation.
- Prevents putrefaction and digestive fermentation.
- Possible weight loss.

5. Animal or plant proteins?

Nutrition is a field in which various dietary philosophies exist side by side, including vegetarianism and the omnivorous diet. Animal products remain essential, in particular for the quality and bioavailability of their proteins, their role in satiety, and their benefits for cellular health.

Proteins are essential macronutrients for building, maintaining and repairing body tissues, as well as for producing enzymes and hormones. The bioavailability of proteins refers to the ease with which our body can digest, absorb and use them.

Animal products, such as meat, fish and eggs, offer complete proteins containing all the essential amino acids that the body cannot produce itself. These proteins are generally easier for our bodies to use than those from plant sources. Studies indicate that animal proteins contribute to a greater feeling of satiety, which can help regulate food intake and maintain a healthy body weight.

In comparison, extracting proteins and essential amino acids from plant sources can be more complex. Plant proteins are often considered incomplete, as they may lack one or more essential amino acids. To obtain a complete amino acid profile from plant foods, it is necessary to consume a variety of plant protein sources, which may require more careful dietary planning.

Animal products provide not only high-quality protein but also other essential nutrients for healthy cell function and construction, such as vitamin B12, haem iron, omega-3s, vitamin D and calcium. These elements play crucial roles in various aspects of health, including red blood cell production, brain health and bone health.

To maximise the benefits of animal products while minimising the potential negative effects, such as the acidity associated with meat consumption, it is advisable to combine them with the right accompaniments, particularly vegetables. Vegetables, rich in fibre and nutrients, can help to regulate acidity and promote better digestion and absorption of nutrients. This approach of balanced food combinations optimises nutritional benefits while supporting overall health.

The consumption of animal products, when integrated into a varied and balanced diet, can play an important role in providing bioavailable proteins and other essential nutrients. However, it is essential to choose quality sources and favour sustainable farming practices to have a positive impact on health and the environment.

6. Are there any deficiencies at the end of a dry fast?

There is a widespread belief that dry fasting could induce nutritional deficiencies due to a temporary decrease in minerals in the body at the end of the practice. However, this perspective does not fully capture the regenerative and rebalancing potential that dry fasting can offer. Although it is true that a slight demineralisation may occur, this phenomenon is not only temporary but also a prelude to a substantial improvement in the individual's nutritional state.

In the weeks following the end of dry fasting, a remarkable phenomenon occurs: the body's capacity to assimilate nutrients increases considerably. Mineral and vitamin reserves, far from remaining depleted, increase fivefold. This amplification is made possible by the reset of the digestive system and the improvement in metabolic efficiency brought about by fasting. In other words, the human body is perfectly equipped to manage the mineral 'debt' imposed by a 12-day dry fast without suffering any lasting damage.

The reintroduction of nutrients post-fasting is crucial to capitalise on this window of hyper-assimilation. Proteins in particular need to be reintroduced quickly to support cellular reconstruction and regeneration. Autophagy processes, stimulated during fasting, continue to eliminate non-functional cells and cellular components, making way for the creation of new bioavailable nutrients.

Clinical studies and blood tests after dry fasting reveal significant improvements in blood composition. Individuals previously deficient in iron saw their levels normalise after just one week of dry fasting. These results suggest that dry fasting, far from inducing deficiencies, may in fact help to correct certain pre-existing nutritional deficiencies.

However, during the transition to a normal diet, it is essential to avoid industrial and acidic foods. Because of their ability to leach minerals from the body, these foods can counteract the benefits gained during fasting. A diet rich in nutrients, favouring natural and whole food sources, is therefore recommended to support and prolong the benefits of dry fasting.

In summary, dry fasting appears not only to be a safe practice in terms of managing nutritional reserves, but also a powerful catalyst for optimising general health. By adopting a cautious and informed approach both during the fast and when food is reintroduced, it is possible to maximise the benefits of this ancient practice, paving the way for improved health and renewed vitality.

CHAPTER 20

Medical indications for dry fasting

1. Depression, anxiety, malaise

Functional disorders of the nervous system, such as depression or anxiety, affect many people, either directly or indirectly. Depression and physical ill-being are characterised by common symptoms: chronic sadness, anxiety, frustration, despair, pessimism, anguish and so on. People may feel guilty, useless, powerless or incapable, losing interest in life and becoming indifferent to activities they once enjoyed. Sleep disorders, obsessions, insomnia or hypersomnia are also common.

The main cause of depression and physical malaise is always the same. It is an endogenous intoxication of the body that leads to high levels of toxins and disrupts all the organs and tissues, as well as all the biochemical processes in the central nervous system. Stress and past traumas return. The difficulty of managing these emotions exacerbates the excessive toxaemia affecting the entire central nervous system.

Dry fasting pushes people to their limits. Faced with a situation of extreme deprivation, the person is bound to break free in one way or another. People turn away from the outside world and concentrate more on nature, beauty, health and the treatment they are undergoing for their health. The body fights for survival. According to the principle of dominance, two types of stress cannot coexist simultaneously in the body: the stronger wins. Dry fasting is a major but controlled stress for the body, controlled by the patient's will and state of mind. This is why all pathological symptoms disappear during dry fasting. Patients develop a strong desire to live, because they are indirectly close to death, and become calmer, kinder and more empathetic when they leave dry fasting.

Our mind and body are closely linked. Quality detoxification, as offered by dry fasting, helps to restore the normal functioning of the intestines and liver and all the other organs, allowing the brain to receive quality nutrition and sufficient quantities of oxygen. Disrupted biochemical processes normalise and improve considerably.

This perspective on depression and its treatment highlights the importance of a holistic approach to health, recognising the complex interaction between mind, body and environment. It also emphasises the power of individual will and self-management in the healing process.

As well as dry fasting, you can use phytotherapy with plants such as valerian, hawthorn and lemon balm. For people wanting to improve their ability to adapt to a difficult situation or people going through a difficult period psychologically, I would add two plants:

- Rhodiola and Ginseng in Quantis, from the lpev.fr lab
- Carry out a one-month course of treatment.

Add magnesium and, of course, a little aromatherapy such as petit grain bigaradier, four drops a day internally or by olfaction.

2. Rheumatic and autoimmune diseases.

Diseases such as rheumatoid arthritis, ankylosing spondylitis, osteoarthritis deformans and infectious polyarthritis represent a major challenge in the healthcare field, due to their chronic and progressive nature. Rheumatoid arthritis, one of the most common joint diseases, mainly affects women and is characterised by chronic inflammation of the joints. Although the exact causes of this disease are still unknown, immunological disorders, in particular the autoimmune process, play a crucial role. Particular attention needs to be paid to the intestine, and porosity needs to be assessed, as well as psychological stress, which needs to be addressed.

Recently, dry fasting has been studied as a potential approach to treating these conditions. Dry fasting is a method of total detoxification, eliminating infections and foreign substances from the body. It has shown promising results, notably in restoring immune system function, strengthening cell barriers and improving blood microcirculation. These effects can have a positive impact on autoimmune diseases and rheumatic pain.

Case studies have shown significant improvements in patients suffering from rheumatoid arthritis after following a long dry fast, but several complete cures of at least seven days will be necessary to have a full causal effect. The fasters reported a reduction in joint pain, a reduction in joint deformity and an improvement in mobility after the cure. In some cases, rheumatoid nodules even disappeared, suggesting that dry fasting could also be beneficial in the treatment of other autoimmune diseases.

Rheumatism can also be exacerbated or triggered by bacterial infections, particularly oral bacteria. The use of medicinal plants such as devil's claw, white willow and ginger can be an effective complementary strategy. Neem is an anti-bacterial that needs to be used for two to three months to have a preparatory effect. These plants have anti-inflammatory and analgesic properties that can relieve pain and reduce inflammation.

In conclusion, dry fasting is emerging as an innovative and powerful approach to the treatment of autoimmune pathologies and rheumatic pain. By combining this method with the use of medicinal plants targeting bacterial causes and relieving pain, it is possible to offer a holistic and effective treatment strategy for these debilitating conditions.

3. Dry fasting and cardiovascular improvement

Before starting a dry fast, it is essential to prepare the body. Physical exercise plays a crucial role in detoxification and improving cardiovascular function. At the same time, a low-carb diet rich in vegetables and animal proteins helps to condition the body for fasting, while contributing to general health.

The use of coenzyme Q10 and magnesium is beneficial for maintaining heart muscle. These dietary supplements support heart function and help prevent cardiovascular disease. Plants such as olive and hawthorn are known for their positive effects on cholesterol and hypertension. They can be incorporated into the diet to boost cardiovascular health.

Dry fasting is particularly effective in cleansing the blood. During dry fasting, the heart loses virtually no weight. Blood circulation in the heart muscle improves and its glycogen reserves increase. There is a marked reduction in heart attacks, necrosis or inflammation of the heart muscle. Heart rate normalises and heart rhythm decreases.

In patients suffering from hypertension, fasting has an immediate effect on blood pressure, which falls within the first few days. After five to seven days of dry fasting, even in patients with persistent, long-term illnesses, blood pressure returns to normal.

After fasting, it is crucial to maintain a healthy diet, low in carbohydrates and rich in vegetables and animal proteins, to prolong the beneficial effects of fasting on the cardiovascular system.

4. Dry fasting and fertility

One of the main benefits of dry fasting is its detoxifying potential. By eliminating toxins accumulated in the body, dry fasting can help to improve general health, which can indirectly influence fertility. Toxins in the body can affect the endocrine system, which is responsible for regulating reproductive hormones. By reducing the toxic load, dry fasting helps to normalise hormonal function, which improves fertility.

Dry fasting also stimulates autophagy, a cell regeneration process in which cells break down and eliminate damaged or unnecessary components. This cellular regeneration can have a positive effect on the reproductive organs, improving their function and potentially increasing the chances of fertility. In addition, better cellular health throughout the body can improve the quality of eggs and sperm, key elements in fertility.

A course of dry fasting can also lead to a general improvement in health, including better weight management, reduced inflammation and improved blood circulation. These effects can contribute to a healthier body environment for conception.

5. Dry fasting and digestive pathologies

Dry fasting has a positive influence on the digestive system. It resets and rejuvenates this system, offering a beneficial break from food processing and the management of digestive disorders of all kinds, often linked to an inadequate diet, stress or a sedentary lifestyle. Fasting reduces digestive inflammation even more effectively than water fasting, improves intestinal health and promotes better absorption of nutrients, thus playing a crucial role in weight management.

Intermittent dry fasting in particular provides periods of rest for the digestive system, reducing intestinal inflammation and improving problems such as bloating and irregular bowel movements, while also having a positive impact on the intestinal microbiome. The duration of fasting varies according to individual needs, with short fasts already bringing positive changes and longer fasts ideal for optimal cellular regeneration.

Fasting also has a beneficial effect on the gastric and duodenal mucosa, reducing symptoms of pain, nausea, heartburn and vomiting. It also improves liver function with a choleretic effect and, of course, helps to detoxify the liver and even dissolve gallstones. The addition of foods rich in natural probiotics during periods of non-fasting supports healthy intestinal function. In short, fasting offers a natural and effective method of restoring and maintaining digestive health, relieving unpleasant symptoms and promoting the regeneration of damaged tissues.

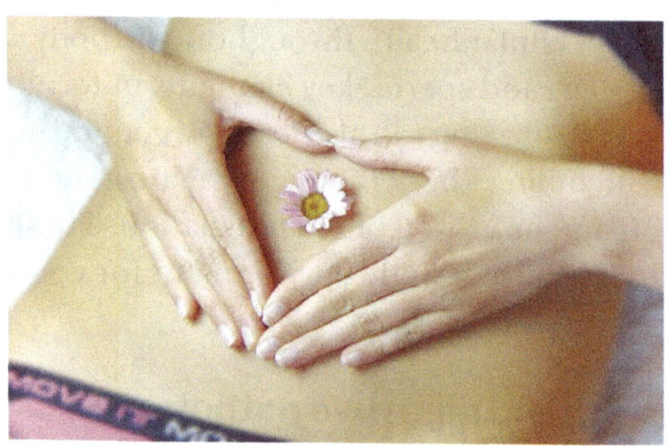

6. Effective treatment of intestinal porosity and associated pathologies

Intestinal porosity, characterised by abnormal permeability of the intestinal barrier, is a pathological condition linked to many diseases, including autoimmune disorders, chronic inflammatory diseases and various gastrointestinal conditions. One of the main advantages of dry fasting is the rest it gives the digestive system. With no food to process, the digestive organs can concentrate on healing and repair. This break reduces the workload on the intestine and allows the intestinal mucosa to regenerate more effectively.

Dry fasting also plays a crucial role in combating inflammation, a key factor in intestinal porosity and associated diseases. By reducing exposure to foods and substances that can cause irritation or inflammation of the intestinal mucosa, fasting helps to calm inflammation and restore a healthy balance in the gastrointestinal tract.

Dry fasting also helps to regulate and calm pathogens in the digestive tract. By reducing the intake of nutrients that can feed bacteria and other harmful micro-organisms, fasting helps to reduce their proliferation and their negative impact on intestinal health.

Another crucial aspect of dry fasting is its ability to stimulate tissue regeneration through the activation of stem cells. During fasting, the body mobilises and utilises its energy reserves, promoting cell regeneration and tissue repair, including damaged intestinal mucosa. This regeneration process plays an essential role in healing intestinal porosity and restoring normal intestinal function.

In short, dry fasting is an effective way of treating intestinal porosity and associated pathologies. By giving the digestive system a rest, combating inflammation, calming pathogens and promoting regeneration of the digestive mucosa through the activation of stem cells, dry fasting helps to restore the integrity and functionality of the intestinal barrier, thereby improving overall health.

7. Treatment of respiratory and infectious diseases using dry fasting

Dry fasting is proving to be an effective and natural method of treating acute infections, particularly respiratory illnesses and influenza. This approach is based on the principle that all inflammation needs liquid to develop and that micro-organisms, such as microbes and viruses, only multiply in sufficiently humid conditions. Dry fasting also increases immunity and fights any infection.

During acute viral infections, characterised by symptoms such as coughing, congested bronchi, runny nose, sore throat and fever, fatigue and pain, the body seeks to detoxify and free itself from excess nutrition and stress. Dry fasting amplifies this process by depriving pathogens of an environment favourable to their growth, thereby reducing inflammation and accelerating healing. It has been observed that inflammatory diseases are treated two to three times faster with dry fasting than with water fasting.

The human body can withstand up to 15 days of water deprivation, during which time microbes die instantly for lack of water. In addition, the body can synthesise water by drawing oxygen from the air and hydrogen from adipose tissue, which explains the rapid weight loss during dry fasting.

Acute respiratory illnesses can be cured in just two to three days, and pneumonia in four to five days with dry fasting. In the case of infectious and respiratory diseases, dry fasting should be started as soon as the first symptoms appear. Immediate cessation of food and water consumption is crucial to stop the infection progressing.

Thanks to its effectiveness in combating inflammation and infections, dry fasting is not limited to the treatment of respiratory diseases, but is also useful for treating various internal or external organ inflammations, including liver and skin disorders. In short, dry fasting is a powerful, natural treatment method for a variety of infectious and respiratory pathologies, offering a fast, effective, free and simple way of restoring human health and well-being.

8. Treatment of bronchopulmonary pathologies and dry fasting

Asthma and bronchopulmonary diseases represent a major challenge for modern medicine. New approaches such as dry fasting, the Buteyko breathing method and the use of natural remedies such as plantain and blackcurrant, as well as sauna treatments, offer promising prospects for the treatment of these conditions. During fasting, the body eliminates accumulated toxins, which can reduce inflammation of the airways and improve breathing in asthma patients.

Buteyko breathing and square breathing are techniques that teach how to control breathing to improve tissue oxygenation and reduce hyperventilation. This method can be particularly beneficial for asthma sufferers, as it helps to regulate breathing and reduce the frequency and severity of asthma attacks. Plants such as plantain and blackcurrant have long been used for their beneficial properties on the respiratory tract. Plantain is known for its expectorant and anti-inflammatory effects, while blackcurrant can help boost the immune system and reduce inflammation of the respiratory tract. Sauna therapy is another therapeutic approach for bronchopulmonary diseases. The heat of the sauna can help relax the muscles of the respiratory tract, reduce inflammation and promote the elimination of toxins through perspiration.

By combining dry fasting, the Buteyko breathing method, the use of medicinal plants and the sauna, patients suffering from asthma and bronchopulmonary diseases can find significant relief and an improvement in their quality of life. However, it is important to consult a healthcare professional before starting any new therapy, in particular to ensure that these methods are suitable for each individual case.

9. Dry fasting and cancer

- **Dry fasting: a global approach to cancer treatment**

It is essential to adopt a holistic strategy to treat cancer, targeting not only the disease itself, but also the underlying causes and the general well-being of the individual. Dry fasting has emerged as a powerful tool in this comprehensive approach to cancer treatment.

- **A success story in cancer treatment**

I remember several people who undertook dry fasts and there was a real stabilisation, even a reset to zero of all health parameters.

Early intervention. If you are inclined to dry fasting, it is ideal to do so before undergoing chemotherapy or radiotherapy. Chemotherapy destroys cells indiscriminately, including immune cells that compromise the body's natural defence mechanisms.

Sustained fasting cures (three per year). It is advisable to undertake a series of fasting cures, incorporating anti-cancer herbs, until the malignant tumour is completely eradicated.

Lifestyle and dietary changes: A complete change of lifestyle and diet is crucial to recovery. This includes moving to environmentally-friendly areas to reduce the immune system's exposure to industrial toxins.

Ongoing preventive measures: Even after successful treatment with dry fasting, lifelong preventive fasting is necessary to avoid recurrence. Unfortunately, this requirement is often unattainable for many patients due to a lack of motivation.

When dry fasting is practised, there is an intense purification of the body, which encourages the rapid emergence of large quantities of natural killers in a state of advanced preparation. This process significantly extends the life of macrophages and other immune system cells. A crucial aspect of this mechanism is the activation of macrophages, making them capable of eliminating atypical malignant cells, while displaying increased cytotoxic activity against any damaged cells. There is also an increase in the production of tumour necrosis factor and interleukins.

Without access to food, phagocytes begin to perform their primary function: capturing and digesting bacteria, viruses, cellular debris and ageing or dying cells, thereby contributing to the renewal and potential rejuvenation of the body. All defective cells, including cancer cells, which are naturally present in the body, are digested. The selection of diseased cells over healthy cells during dry fasting is also due to the expulsion of lympho-epithelial cells from the entire digestive tract.

As body temperature rises, metabolic processes intensify, accelerating the destruction of cells, including cancer cells. The effectiveness of T lymphocytes, essential in this process, is optimised by a high temperature. Studies have shown that increasing the temperature of tumours can reduce their size, making it easier for the immune system to seek out and eliminate foreign and modified elements.

A tumour cannot grow beyond the size of a pinhead without an autonomous blood supply. Angiogenesis, by supplying oxygen and nutrients, is essential to tumour growth and spread. Dry fasting thickens the blood, particularly in pathologically altered areas, slowing the development of blood vessels within the tumour and damaging its blood and nutrient supply. This inhibits tumour growth and can lead to the degeneration of large masses, giving them a soft, gelatinous consistency, eventually leading to their disappearance.

This therapeutic framework triggered by dry fasting is essential for autolysis. Studies suggest that in a context of artificially restricted intake, cancer cells, which are highly dependent on surrounding tissues for their survival, often die. Because of their rapid growth, these cells require substantial quantities of nutrients, far in excess of the needs of normal cells. Obesity and an unhealthy diet are known to increase the risk of cancer.

It is essential to integrate targeted biotherapies into cancer treatment, requiring a holistic approach to maximise efficacy. Fasting cures lasting at least nine days can be envisaged to cut metastases, thereby enriching the strategies for combating this disease. To this day, dry fasting remains a first-level therapy that should be used as soon as possible in the early stages of cancer. The chances of success are very high.

- **Addressing holistic needs in cancer treatment**

In addition to dry fasting, several other aspects are crucial in the treatment of cancer:

Emotional well-being: Taking emotional aspects into account, understanding past traumas and integrating psycho-corporal therapies is essential.

Dietary changes: Changing your diet to make it less inflammatory and incorporating effective supplements can have a significant impact on healing.

Detoxification: Regular detoxification of the body, focusing particularly on the liver and intestines, is vital.

Food supplements and specific plants. All naturopaths should have everything they need on their palette to achieve a powerful therapeutic effect.

Short and long dry fasts: Both short and long dry fasts, when properly monitored, can significantly improve the chances of successful treatment.

Solutions in Oncology and for Autoimmune Diseases

Cancer is a complex and multifactorial disease that requires a holistic approach for optimal management. While conventional treatments such as surgery, chemotherapy, and radiotherapy remain essential according to your doctor, many people turn to natural solutions to complement these treatments or choose an entirely different path.

Lifestyle Hygiene

Lifestyle hygiene plays a crucial role in the prevention and management of cancer. Adopting healthy habits can help strengthen the immune system and reduce risk factors.

- **Avoid Tobacco and Alcohol**: These substances are known carcinogens.

- **Reduce Exposure to Environmental Toxins**: Minimize exposure to industrial chemicals and pesticides.
- **Hydration**: Drink enough water to help flush toxins from the body.

Sleep

Sleep is essential for cellular regeneration and overall health. Quality sleep allows the body to repair damage and strengthen the immune system.

- **Sleep Routine**: Maintain a regular sleep routine by going to bed and waking up at the same time each day.
- **Sleep Environment**: Create a conducive sleep environment that is dark and quiet.

Keto Diet

The ketogenic diet, high in fats and low in carbohydrates, can be beneficial for cancer patients by limiting the availability of glucose, the primary fuel for cancer cells.

- **Recommended Foods**: Avocados, nuts, seeds, healthy oils, low-carb vegetables, and lean meats.
- **Avoid**: Sugars, grains, and high-carb fruits.

Dietary Supplements

Dietary supplements can provide additional support by supplying essential nutrients and boosting immune defences.

- **Vitamins and Minerals**: Vitamin D, Vitamin C, zinc, and selenium.
- **Antioxidants**: Curcumin, resveratrol, and green tea extracts.

Pine Resin

Pine resin, particularly from balsam fir, is known for its antiseptic and anti-inflammatory properties. It can be used for its potential benefits in managing cancer symptoms and underlying causes.

Physical Exercise

Regular physical activity is beneficial for improving the quality of life of cancer patients and can help reduce the side effects of treatments.

- **Types of Exercises**: Walking, yoga, tai chi, and resistance exercises.
- **Benefits**: Improved strength, endurance, mood, and reduced fatigue.

Medicinal Mushrooms

Medicinal mushrooms have been used for centuries in traditional medicine for their immunomodulatory and anticancer properties. Use these under the guidance of a healthcare practitioner.

- **Coriolus versicolor (Turkey Tail)**: Contains polysaccharides that can stimulate the immune system.
- **Reishi (Ganoderma lucidum)**: Known for its immunostimulant and anti-inflammatory properties.
- **Chaga (Inonotus obliquus)**: Recognized for its antioxidant effects and immune support.
- **Cordyceps**: Improves energy, endurance, and possesses immunomodulatory properties.

Therapeutic Dry Fasting

- **Regular Short Fasts**: Fasting for 16 to 24, or 36 hours once a week can help improve insulin sensitivity, reduce inflammation, and stimulate autophagy, a cellular cleaning process that is very helpful in oncology.
  - **Practice**: Choose one or two days a week to fast for 16 to 24 hours, drinking only water, tea, or unsweetened coffee.

  - **Benefits**: Stimulates cell repair, improves immune response, and reduces oxidative stress.
- **Long Sequenced Fasts (five to ten days every three months)**: This type of fasting works on the overall health and underlying causes. It can help reset the immune system and should be done with the guidance of a trained professional.
  - **Practice**: Perform prolonged fasts every few weeks or months, ensuring good hydration between dry fasts and consuming electrolytes if necessary.
  - **Benefits**: Reduces insulin and IGF-1 levels (insulin-like growth factor), decreases systemic inflammation, and enhances resistance to chemotherapy treatments if taken.

Mindset

A positive mindset and stress management are essential for fighting cancer and other diseases.

- **Stress Management Techniques**: Meditation, deep breathing, and positive visualization.
- **Emotional Support**: Therapy, support groups, and discussions with loved ones.

Integrating natural solutions into cancer management can provide valuable support to conventional treatments. A holistic approach, combining lifestyle hygiene, sleep, ketogenic diet, dietary supplements, pine resin, physical exercise, medicinal mushrooms, fasting, and a positive mindset, can help improve the quality of life and well-being of cancer patients. It is essential to consult healthcare professionals before implementing these strategies to ensure their compatibility with ongoing treatments. Other effective natural care methods exist, but in such cases, it is best to be accompanied in a professional setting.

CHAPTER 21

Beliefs about dry fasting

- **Belief No. 1: Dehydration leads to rapid death.**

Without water, survival is limited to two to three days. Severe dehydration occurs after 30-40 hours and vital functions deteriorate in 50-60 hours. Without water, symptoms include hallucinations, loss of consciousness and intense headaches.

The realities of dry fasting: Water represents around 70% of the human body mass. During a dry fast, the body produces around 400ml of water per day, mainly through the oxidation of fat. This internal metabolic water production increases significantly, meeting the body's needs for a certain period. In addition, the body stores water under the skin (up to two litres) and in certain cavities (serous cavities). For example, a 60kg person could have more than 30 litres of water in their body.

The body's capacity to adapt: Physiologically, a body undergoing dry fasting does not experience a substantial liquid deficit. Each kilogram of body fat or glycogen releases up to one litre of endogenous metabolic water per day. Fluid loss through perspiration and evaporation is 1.5 to two litres per day. This means that the water deficit does not exceed 0.5 to one litre per day, which is physiologically acceptable.

Anecdotes and studies: There are documented cases of people surviving without water for prolonged periods. For example, a boy survived 13 days under rubble after an earthquake in Mexico in 1985, and Andreas Mihavecz, an 18-year-old Austrian, survived 18 days in a detention cell without water in 1979. Even a dog stayed alive for 103 days without food after an earthquake. These cases demonstrate that the body can resist longer than the three days often quoted, especially in the absence of panic and stress. Many positive testimonials from people who have fasted for between seven and ten days with great benefits are available on my Youtube channel "Therapeutic dry fasting - Michel Deladoey".

Belief no. 2: Dry fasting could worsen the condition of the kidneys.
Response:
There are a number of factors related to diet, sedentary lifestyle and mental health that can adversely affect kidney health.

- Power supply.
- Too much salt: Consuming too much salt can increase blood pressure, which can damage the kidneys.
- Protein-rich foods: Excessive consumption of protein, particularly of animal origin, can increase the workload on the kidneys and lead to long-term damage.
- Processed foods rich in phosphorus: A high intake of phosphorus, often found in processed foods, can be harmful to the kidneys, especially in those who already have kidney disease.
- Sedentary lifestyle.
- Lack of exercise: A sedentary lifestyle increases the risk of illnesses such as hypertension and diabetes, major risk factors for kidney disease.
- Mental health.
- Stress and somatisation: Chronic stress can have a negative impact on overall health and contribute to problems such as hypertension, a risk factor for kidney disease.

- Fear and anxiety: Anxiety can lead to behaviours that are harmful to kidney health, such as poor diet or lack of exercise.
- Water quality and kidney health: The quality of drinking water is crucial to kidney health. Poor-quality water, whether chlorinated or lacking in trace elements, can affect the kidneys.

Effects of dry fasting on the kidneys: Dry fasting can give the kidneys and liver a rest, allowing them to recover more quickly. Studies indicate changes in urine during dry fasting, with subsequent normalisation. In certain kidney diseases, dry fasting has shown positive results, reducing inflammation and normalising urinary composition.

Scientific study: A 2013 German study suggests that dry fasting improves kidney function, even after five days. This study published on PubMed reinforces the idea that dry fasting can be beneficial for the kidneys.

Conclusion: Dry fasting, if properly prepared and carried out, can have a positive effect on kidney function. It is essential to consult a health professional before undertaking dry fasting, especially if pre-existing medical problems are present.

Link to the study: https://pubmed.ncbi.nlm.nih.gov/24434757/

- **Belief no. 3 Dry fasting is a major source of stress and is anti-physiological.**

Response:

Dry fasting is often seen as a potential source of stress for the body. But let's look at what an injured animal does in the wild. It practises dry fasting and waits for its health to improve. However, it is important to consider that the stress factors in our daily lives, such as poor lifestyle, lack of physical activity, difficult relationships and unbalanced diet, can have a much more significant impact on our health than dry fasting itself. It's also worth noting that the more you fast, the less complicated it will be.

In reality, dry fasting, when practised appropriately and under supervision, may not be a major source of stress for the body. On the contrary, it can provide a time of rest and recuperation, of cleansing, allowing the body to concentrate on detoxification and regeneration processes. Dry fasting should be approached with caution, taking into account the individual's state of health.

On the other hand, daily lifestyle stressors have a much more direct and ongoing impact on our well-being. A poor diet, rich in processed foods, sugar and saturated fats, can lead to a range of health problems, including obesity, cardiovascular disease and diabetes. Lack of physical activity contributes to a sedentary lifestyle, which is a major risk factor for many chronic diseases. Conflicting personal relationships and a stressful environment at work or at home can also lead to mental health problems, such as anxiety and depression.

In conclusion, although dry fasting requires a cautious and informed approach, it is essential to recognise that the stress factors associated with everyday life have a much greater impact on our health.

- **Belief no. 4: Nutritional deficiencies**

Many nutritionists claim that during fasting there is a vitamin deficiency because the body does not receive any proteins or fats.

During dry fasting, you consume the structural proteins in your own tissues. Vitamin deficiencies do not occur with dry fasting. This is where nutritionists start talking about the possibility of vitamin deficiency with prolonged dry fasting. And this is supposedly because of a simple analogy: if, they say, a diet with a lack of minerals, trace elements and vitamins causes vitamin deficiency, then dry fasting should lead to it all the more.

In fact, however, the opposite is true. With therapeutic dry fasting, the body does not expend energy on digestion, assimilation and excretion. At the same time, mineral requirements are considerably reduced and the body uses its available reserves much more economically. As a result, vitamin deficiencies are very often observed with mono-food or unbalanced diets that result in the loss of all minerals, when refined and denatured foods are used.

In dry fasting, reserves are redistributed and the release of toxins and the proper functioning of the organs allow increased release and availability of micronutrients in the body.

Anaemia, for example, is easily treated by one or two courses of long-term dry fasting. The famous American researcher Dr Vies wrote: "*You can live longer by fasting on water rather than on water and white flour, simply because eating white flour increases the need for other substances for the body to digest, absorb and metabolise the flour*". Nutritionists say: "*Without proteins during fasting, the body, in addition to fats, consumes the structural proteins of its own tissues*". The evolutionary acquisitions that increase animals' chances of survival in the absence of food include the internal food supply. These are calorie-rich lipids dissolved in body fluids, liver glycogen, muscle glycogen and specialised cells. Adipose tissue and its cells, the adipocytes, are rich in fat and are the carriers of living energy. During the period of growth with a well-nourished life, their number increases. During fasting, they become an internal source of nutrition. Live storage cells are an excellent dietary programme solution. Think about how you can try to keep food warm in a healthy and inexpensive way!

During fasting, adipocytes supply the body not only with energy, but also with almost all the components necessary for life. A person who fasts does not suffer from malnutrition. One kilogram of adipose tissue is enough for five days of good nutrition! Even people of ideal weight have adipose tissue. Dry fasting has two very big plus points: less muscle tissue is lost than fat. During dry fasting, fat tissue breaks down three to four times faster than muscle tissue, because fat tissue is more than 90% water and muscle tissue remains relatively intact.

One hundred years ago, on the basis of extensive research, the academician V.V. Pashutin discovered that pathologically altered tissues are consumed during fasting. It is the liberation of the body from old, diseased, dead, weak, flaccid and decaying cells and tissues that determines a powerful therapeutic effect in a variety of diseases. After all, not only do the healthy tissues not suffer, but they are renewed, so to speak, resulting in the rejuvenating effect noted by all researchers, ancient and modern. All the vital organs, the heart, the central nervous system, the brain, the endocrine glands, during therapeutic fasting, however long it lasts, maintain their condition and are even considerably improved. These are the factors which explain the phenomena during therapeutic dry fasting, such as the increase in creative capacities in brain workers, writers, musicians, inventors and artists. Their performance increases immeasurably, consciousness becomes clearer, the quality of thought improves: it deepens, the circle of associations widens considerably, long-term and short-term memory improves, and so on.

To criticise and reject the therapeutic dry fasting method, you first need to be competent in this field, and to study and experiment with it. Without this, any criticism of dry fasting is totally unfounded. Dry fasting is part of nature and has been part of our genetic programme for millions of years. Animals that are sick in the wild and isolated do not need a doctor: dry fasting is their first therapy.

Belief no. 5: The Power of Dry Fasting in the Healing of Diseases
Many people believe that dry fasting is a panacea, capable of curing all illnesses, including stage four cancers. Although this method has shown remarkable effectiveness in various cases, it is essential to understand its limitations and appropriate applications.

Effectiveness in Inflammatory Processes: Dry fasting excels particularly in the treatment of inflammation. It is effective not only for colds, but also for inflammation of the internal and external organs, such as skin boils, inflammation of the inner ear, bruising and various infections. However, it does not directly heal bone fractures, although it can speed up the resolution of the associated oedema and inflammation.

Therapeutic complements: Adding therapies such as Metatron or Triomed bioresonance can increase the effectiveness of dry fasting.

Post-concussion use: Preventive post-concussion dry fasting helps to control swelling of brain tissue, promoting faster recovery.

Effects on serious illnesses: In severe illnesses such as rheumatoid arthritis, osteoarthritis, fibromyalgia, autoimmune disorders and cancer, prolonged dry fasting for seven to 11 days has been shown to be very effective. It can also help dissolve ovarian cysts and make benign tumours disappear.

Limitations and complications: This method is often adopted at a late stage, after the failure of conventional treatments and drug abuse, when the patient's vitality is already diminished. The body, weakened by medication, radiation and reduced natural defences, may not respond as effectively to dry fasting. Serious complications can arise, especially without professional guidance.

Experiences in my practice: I have helped people in the initial stages of their disease through several cycles of dry fasting and a complete change of lifestyle. On the other hand, patients who had undergone chemotherapy or radiotherapy and had fasted at home did not achieve the same results.

Misunderstanding and prejudice: Dry fasting is often misunderstood and unfairly blamed. Terminally ill patients may die during fasting, but the cause is the illness itself, not the fasting.

Similarly, people with heart disease die after heavy meals, but this does not imply that fasting is to blame. Fasting is a digestive rest and a pathway to life, but misunderstandings and the limits of our understanding can lead to erroneous conclusions.

CHAPTER 22

Testimonies and clinical cases of dry fasting

1. Clinical cases

- **Bernard 52 years old**

Medical history: Mild hypertension, overweight, sleep apnoea.

Bernard suffered from moderate sleep apnoea and intense snoring which disrupted his sleep and that of his partner. He had tried several methods to improve his sleep quality, including the use of a CPAP machine and lifestyle changes, but without significant success.

He began with short 24-hour fasting periods, which he gradually increased to 48 hours once a month. During these periods, he consumed neither food nor water. Then he did a five-day dry fast, which was very effective.

Bernard kept a diary detailing his experience of dry fasting, including his physical and mental sensations. In the first few weeks, he noticed a slight improvement in his sleep and a reduction in snoring. After three months of regular dry fasting and his five-day dry fast, Bernard noticed a significant improvement in the quality of his sleep. His snoring had completely disappeared, and he felt more rested when he woke up.

Results: Six months after starting dry fasting, Bernard underwent a new polysomnography. The results showed a remarkable reduction in sleep apnoea episodes and a general improvement in the quality of his sleep. In addition, Bernard lost weight and his blood pressure stabilised.

Conclusion: Dry fasting had a positive impact on Bernard's quality of sleep, eliminating his snoring and reducing the symptoms of his sleep apnoea. These changes contributed to an overall improvement in his well-being and health.

- **Sidonie**

62-year-old woman cured by long dry fasting.

Medical history: Chronic arthritis, inflammation of the joints of the hands, high levels of C-reactive protein (CRP) indicating systemic inflammation.

Intervention: Two cures of dry fasting, each lasting eight days, with an interval of six months between the two.

Results of the first treatment:

- Significant improvement in hand joint deformity.
- Reduced pain and joint stiffness.
- Inflammation markers, particularly CRP, showed a downward trend.

Results after six months and the second treatment:

- Stabilisation of the improvement in joint deformity observed after the first treatment.
- Normalisation of CRP levels, indicating a reduction in systemic inflammation.
- General improvement in well-being, energy and mobility.

Conclusion: Dry fasting had a positive impact on arthritis symptoms and inflammatory markers in this patient. Repeating the treatment after six months helped to consolidate the benefits obtained and improve the patient's quality of life.

- **Clinical cases of Lyme disease**
- **Loïc's recovery – Lyme disease and chronic fatigue**

I recovered after four cures of dry fasting lasting ten days. I no longer have any pain or tiredness, which I'd had for years. Dry fasting is an extremely effective therapy for Lyme disease and other infections that I recommend to everyone.
https://www.youtube.com/watch?v=W4ucKTg6g3o&t=1521s

- **Elisa cure – Lyme disease**

I did three consecutive dry fasts over one year because I'd been suffering from Lyme disease for years. To date, I am completely cured following these three long dry fasts. I left a testimonial on Michel's channel.
https://www.youtube.com/watch?v=diAIr_pbbxY&list=UULFlinnpuUQ6agdn9RnmP1DbQ&index=74
Thérèse SCHLUTER

2. Testimonials

- **Interview with Cédric Abeck, director of the international Colife yoga school in Geneva/Switzerland.**

Fasting has always been a process imbued with mystery and revelation, a personal quest towards a better understanding of one's body and mind. My own expedition into the world of dry fasting turned out to be an unexpected adventure, illuminated by the collective strength of a group and the serenity offered by mountainous nature, far from the hustle and bustle of urban life. This adventure, orchestrated by Michel, an experienced guide specialising in dry fasting and naturopathy, was a revelation.

My first long dry fast was an incredible experience. Technically, the first three days were the most arduous, both physically and emotionally. However, despite this turbulence, a constant energy flowed through me, testifying to the body's surprising ability to adapt to the absence of food and energy.

I was even able to teach yoga and walk for four hours in the mountains on the sixth day. The group experience proved crucial. Together, time seemed to expand differently, passing with a speed that contrasted with the slowness of the days of solitary fasting. The exchanges, the sharing of emotions and the mutual support made each stage more accessible, each moment lighter. Initial fears, particularly of not being able to sleep, gradually dissipated in the warmth of the community.

From the fourth day onwards, a threshold seemed to have been crossed. I felt a new assurance that I could continue, strengthened by the trials I had already overcome. Each passing day strengthened my resolve and amazed me at my body's endurance, capable of moving and functioning without the need for external food or water. The ego attacks, recurrent and profound, revealed the layers of my inner self, often prey to childish rebellions and emotional overjections. One evening, for example, the accumulated frustration exploded in a storm of tears, an emotional catharsis that purified my mind and opened my heart. The return to normality, symbolised by the resumption of water consumption, instantly brought back old patterns of thought and judgement. Yet the fast left an indelible mark: a deep physical and mental connection, a reset that took me back, with renewed vigour, to my younger years. The rest of my dry fasts, now more powerful, are rooted in a reality where preparation and collective goodwill are essential. It's not so much the search for an extreme experience that guides my steps, but a quiet commitment to a natural and profoundly transformative process.

Trust, dare to try it without judgement, go slowly – these are the tips I'm sharing today, based on my experience of dry fasting, a practice that goes far beyond simple abstinence to touch the very essence of being.

- **Therapeutic dry fasting cure in Champery, 2023**

I took part in the therapeutic dry fasting cure in Champery (Switzerland) from 22 June to 9 July 2023, accompanied by Michel Deladoey, naturopath, and Marie-Christine Thomas, life coach. At no time did I doubt this healing method, because it's the body's vital force that heals. The group was made up of 18 people from different backgrounds with the same objective: healing and health. There was great solidarity and cohesion between all the members of the group. The sensation of thirst and the disappearance of hunger appeared on the second day. That's when it was important not to break down. I started the therapy with cold water at 11 degrees, which boosted my body. I had a difficult passage from the second to the third day. The symptoms were slight dizziness and a drop in energy. The call to drink was felt, but the need for food had completely disappeared.

My mouth became pasty and I had difficulty speaking from the fourth day onwards. I felt very tired, my body temperature rose and I slept for just a few hours. I could feel my body shrinking from the inside. Without drinking, I continued to urinate every day, because 1kg of fat corresponds to around 800g of water. The body's intelligence manufactures metabolic water.

On the sixth day, Michel asked me to stop the dry fast because my blood pressure was too low and I felt dizzy standing up. The first sip of water I drank was a divine, even ecstatic moment. The post-cure benefits include renewed vital energy six months later, less joint pain in my right knee, less craving for sugar and the disappearance of spots on my face. I had some itching in my stomach which has disappeared. I feel a deep need for a second cure in 2024 in this same place, full of vitality and energy. During these timeless days, I had an extraordinary experience, discovering beautiful people in these magnificent surroundings. I touched the gates of hell and heaven!

Deep gratitude to Michel, tireless researcher and heartfelt thanks to Marie-Christine, exceptional life coach who always listens with kindness and bravo to all the companions on this inner journey.

Therese Schlutter

I took part in the dry fasting cure in Montenegro, a place full of energy, in September 2023 with Michel Deladoey and Marie Christine Thomas, the guides. Thank you both for your guidance and kindness, which went beyond my expectations. After many years of practising water fasting, it was only natural that I should turn to dry fasting to go further with confidence, already convinced of the many benefits of this practice. I also read Michel's book carefully before setting off on this wonderful human adventure... The group of 16 beautiful people was magnificent, rich in support, listening, sharing, solidarity and love. I really felt at home. Which is really important during a dry fasting cure. I never felt hungry. Thirst became a bit more difficult in the middle of the week... and my mouth became very pasty after five days and I didn't feel like talking after seven days. But there were no particular symptoms, just an increase in my body temperature and a physical weakness that didn't stop me from doing yoga every morning and meditating in the evenings, which was a real pleasure. A real feeling of pleasure and renewed Energy with the cold water affusions, below 11 degrees, a real joy. I'd say the hardest part was the night. I slept very little, about two hours, and the night was long. I had to stop my fasting on the eighth day, following the news of the death of my best friend, and that was a huge thank you to Marie-Christine for her support.

Taking another sip of water is fabulous, it's so good. The same goes for the first foods. Having been used to water fasting, I'd say without hesitation that dry fasting is easier and more effective.

The post-dry fasting experience has given me a wonderful energy that continues well into the future, with profound dietary changes, self-examination and the disappearance of addictions... Emotionally, it's been a revelation, I've lived alongside the light and the dark... I've learnt to open my heart... and I'm determined to continue this wonderful journey, which is far from over. I'll be back to deal with some chronic problems in April 2024 and continue my journey towards the light, towards unconditional love. GRATITUDE TO LIFE

Thank you to me for daring to do it, I feel stronger now that I've entered 'another world' where anything is possible...

Babeth

- **Catherine – 78 years old, France. First seven-day dry fasting cure with Michel Deladoey.**

I had already done a water fasting cure with Dr Vivini 50 years ago. When I heard about dry fasting, it reminded me of Dr Ohsawa's macrobiotic movement, which also advocated not drinking if you were ill and that this encouraged faster recovery.

I found it a thousand times more pleasant than the water fast and the symptoms were less severe. After this dry fast, I feel in excellent shape, I walked for two hours yesterday with 300 metres of ascent. I've reaped several benefits from this cure, starting with my skin. I had a wart, which is now going away and I feel younger. What's more, I'm in great spirits now. I came in with a torticollis that started during the confinement and wouldn't go away. I had sciatica. All that went away during the dry fast.

During dry fasting, you don't eat any food, liquid or solid, and you don't think about it any more, unlike water fasting where you try to compensate for the lack of food with water. I found the group very supportive and I learnt a lot about myself and in general during those 15 days.

I really enjoyed the accompanying therapies, the yoga and the ito thermie, which warmed me up. The Schuman plateau also made me feel really good. The secret to a successful dry fasting cure is to trust your therapist. In any case, it was a great experience for me and I'm thinking of coming back next year.

- **Katia – Italy. Nine days of dry fasting**

I took part in a dry fasting retreat in Switzerland, led by Michel Deladoey. I've been suffering from various chronic illnesses for about 30 years. During the consultation, I was advised to do nine days of dry fasting, with a second fast if necessary. I went to Switzerland after having done two preparatory fasts of three days and with some doubts about my ability to last nine days. I immediately understood the importance of doing a dry fast with the support of a competent therapist who assesses and supports the various important stages of the process. Equally important is the support of the group, as we go through different phases together. I was struck by the state of well-being and strength you acquire. Movement becomes almost a necessity for the body (we walked 6-8 km until the seventh day). The purity of the environment is essential, because as we progress, we realise how much we are in a relationship with the environment, how much we exchange and how much we absorb. From the fifth day onwards, the urine monitoring method becomes interesting. It's incredible to see the amount of waste that comes out. You mustn't underestimate the need to resume eating: the continuation of the fasting effect depends on it. I was able to fast for nine days and have a good dietary recovery. Now that the 14-day cure is over, I can say that I feel less burdened, clear-headed and my body feels stronger. It was an unforgettable experience.

- **Lucienne – France – nine days of dry fasting**

This wonderful adventure is coming to an end. These 15 days will remain an extraordinary experience for me. First of all, personally, with this journey to the very depths of my being, and this extraordinary rebirth. The idyllic setting was of paramount importance. The group we formed was a fabulous support, but above all, your guidance gave this adventure an incredible dimension. Your simplicity, Michel, your gentleness but also your rigour, it took a lot to reframe the mischievous and talkative chicks for 15 days. And your professionalism kept me going despite the suffering. I never doubted thanks to the total confidence you inspire. Thank you, thank you for all that and so much more. I'm leaving this morning with a little phrase that came to me during a sleepless night, after I'd started eating again. I touched the gates of hell, and the gates of heaven opened. And I remember a few lines from a poem during one of my love affairs. Let yourself be embraced by the love that burns in you, and your soul escape from the tiny cocoon where it had been confined for so long, forgetting that its world was the firmament. This day, my soul came out of the cocoon. Thank you for life. Lulu.

- **Selena**

My name is Selena and I became interested in dry fasting to improve my health. I did my first eight-day dry fast. It revealed problems with my liver. When I came out of the fast, I had lots of energy and a very good mood. My sleep was improved and I slept longer. My digestive system also improved. I also had athlete's foot which disappeared completely at the end of the eight days.

- **Mario**

My name is Mario. I'm 70 years old and I've finished my ten days of dry fasting. Today I'm on Day 7 of the adapted refeeding My mood has really improved. I'm much more positive than before and I feel completely detoxified both physically and mentally. I look forward to seeing more results over the next two months.

- **Maria**

I came to do a long dry fasting retreat for problems of fibromyalgia that I've had for 30 years, as well as a pituitary adenoma. I'm on my fifth day of refeeding and I've quickly seen the results, because now I can move and walk without pain, whereas before that was impossible for me. I think dry fasting is one of the best treatments for removing all the pain in the body.

- **Alex**

Although I'm physically fit, health is a natural thing and in my opinion, dry fasting is the best way to maintain your health over the long term. I do a preventive cure of seven to ten days a year.

- **Mariana**

Marvellous nature! Therapeutic dry fasting is an experience that's impossible to describe! The body is reborn at the cellular level. You can feel the magic of nature here. For me, after this experience, I can say that dry fasting is the best way to regenerate your health.

This ten-day dry fasting experience is my second. For me, it's much more than a discovery, because not only have I improved my health, but it's much more than that, because I feel like a new person. For those who want to purify themselves and get to know themselves better, dry fasting in the great outdoors will remain an experience that changed my life.

- **Louis**

I'm appealing to those who have launched dry fasting and the technique of healing through abstinence from food and water. I'm 45 years old, I'm skinny and I don't have any particularly serious illnesses, but I still complain a bit about everything, with minor aches and pains. I used the classic water fasting method. It's a long process, but I can't see any results. Then I used the healing method of dry abstinence for just three3 days, and the results were obvious: the joints in my elbow stopped hurting, there was a lightness in my body, a cheerfulness, an optimism. I'd like to fully apply this method for spiritual and physical recovery.

- **Tatiana**

In September 2019, I took part in a nine-day dry fast. It was an unforgettable experience physically and mentally, a time full of emotions and unforgettable scenery and nature that I still carry in my heart. Needless to say, it takes time and determination. You have to keep trying until the fasting technique becomes familiar to you. The psychological support of a group where everyone commits to fasting is stimulating and supportive. During the fast, you achieve a state of physical and mental well-being, a feeling of euphoria, lucidity, concentration and awareness. Once the fast is over, a "nostalgia" is born, a desire to repeat it for the well-being you have felt.

- **Nina**

I was diagnosed with breast cancer three months ago. I didn't want to have the operation, because for some reason I was sure I'd find another way. And the Lord heard me! Friends advised me to do dry fasting. I gathered up my courage and went hungry for three, then seven and finally nine days. You've no idea how I felt at the check-up. And here's the result – the doctors couldn't believe it! The tumour has just disappeared! Dissolved! I bow my head before you, and I'd like to thank you so much for my life and that of my daughter! I know that you have already helped many people to get rid of frightening diagnoses. If only everyone, like me, could overcome my fear and believe in myself and my strength! God bless you! Thank you again!!! Day 8 is the day of liberation. Good mood, a feeling of rebirth! In this day and age, we need to change our whole way of life, and we're already there. I'm very happy with the application of the dry fasting technique.

- **Nicoletta, nine days of dry fasting, Hepatitis C cured**

Hi Michel, I hope all is well.

I've just received the results of the blood tests and ...

There are no more traces of the HCV virus!!!

I'm incredulous, moved, confused, happy and still.

The GOT, GPT and Alfafetoproteins values are a bit high, but I think it's for the regeneration of liver cells that's taking place. I can tell you that up until 22 November I was in great shape and very strong. Since 23 November and for about three days, I've been very tired, without strength, feeling generally unwell and needing a lot of sleep.

I've regained my strength and I feel fine during the day, then towards evening (4/17.00 pm) I feel unwell as if I had a fever: headache (forehead), aching bones and joints, tiredness and sleepiness. I think it's my body working to rebuild itself. I'm in good spirits and have lots of plans. I sleep well and a lot and I have lots of dreams. I still have to come down to earth and realise what a "miracle" this is, but it's certain that I owe you and the whole team a great deal of gratitude, admiration and respect for the help and support you've given me. THANK YOU

- **Jonathan, 52, nine days of dry fasting following a Long Covid and vaccination problem**

I was vaccinated during the Covid period in 2020 and a few days later I developed a Long Covid where I had breathing problems and chronic fatigue which appeared right behind with brain fog, spasms and generalised muscle pain. My vitality level before the Long Covid was ten out of ten and afterwards three out of ten. I'd heard about Michel and dry fasting and that it was supposed to do a complete cellular reset, which I really needed. So, I embarked on a long cure with good preparation. The cure went well in the ideal location of Montenegro and everything was perfect for me with the great people I met. When I came out of the dry fast, I noticed that I was less tired and, above all, that my brain fog had disappeared. What a miracle! A few weeks later, I'm 90% back to health and I'm thinking of doing dry fasting again in six months' time to consolidate my health. This method should be spread everywhere as it would help many people who have been in therapeutic limbo for years without any solutions.

Testimonial from Catherine, aged 60, first dry fast.

Testimony given on her ninth day of dry fasting. She finished her ten days without eating or drinking.

I feel very much alive, I'm very much alive. I miss the water a little and I feel really good. I can see that I'm reaping the benefits of this dry fast and I say to myself why break this dry fast now for a bit of water and to eat. Given that I have the after-effects of Lyme disease and osteoarthritis. Before this dry fast, I was in a lot of pain, but now I'm pain-free. I can say that I'm already feeling an improvement. Of course, I still feel a bit of pain, but it's not like before. My aim was to come here. What medicine hasn't been able to resolve, namely my Lyme and my osteoarthritis, I'm counting on dry fasting to repair. I've read Michel Deladoey's book, which explains that a single dry fast won't solve everything in one go. Sometimes you need two or three dry fasts to improve your health, but it depends on the pathology. I really believe in this method because I feel good. I feel so good that my vital signs are perfect and I've decided to go for nine days. But as Michel says, everyone respects each other and whether you do two, four or six days, it doesn't matter because everyone listens to each other. I feel very well supported by Michel and Marie Christine. The physical and mental aspects of this retreat are completely taken care of, and that's a plus. There are workshops on site, self-care systems and masseuses. I do the Schuman plateau three times a day because Michel told me it was really good for me. The group aspect is also important. Without the group I wouldn't have got this far. Thanks to the group, thanks to the synergy, thanks to the guides, I'm here on a new path of dry fasting. I felt 100% safe in this group and, as you're always meeting people, you never feel alone on this retreat.

Nathalie, four days of dry fasting with Michel Deladoey for the first time in Costa Brava 2024. Testimonial after three days of eating again.

I didn't really know what to expect when I came here because I wasn't very prepared, but I seized the opportunity of a place at the last minute.

When I arrived, I found a really warm group and attentive supervision, offering preventive health systems: Schumann tray, therapeutic blankets, chi machine, massages, yoga.

Initially, I thought I wanted to do a lot more, but I came up against reality. What I appreciate about these cures is the great freedom they offer, where each person evolves according to their own personality. What's particularly remarkable is the gradual and collective return to eating. I have to say that I felt completely safe during this fast. I appreciated the human warmth and the technical, psychological and emotional support. I found it very important and comprehensive.

I also noticed a clear difference between the highly prepared participants and those with less experience, but I'm very glad I did it. Fasting isn't really taught and there are a lot of fears about it. There's always this idea of listening to your body while fasting and not becoming fasting extremists, because each metabolism works at its own pace.

Finally, I'm very happy to have discovered so many things and met so many wonderful people. The people who come to these cures have a certain self-awareness and are open to experience before passing judgement, and that's fundamental.

I have to say that the pain in my hands has disappeared and my tinnitus has virtually stopped. Marie-Christine gave us emotional tools to manage ourselves better and become autonomous. Understanding what we're doing is crucial in fasting in order to achieve the greatest possible autonomy.

- **Many testimonials on my YouTube channel – jeune sec thérapeutique – Michel Deladoey**

Anna's Dry Fasting Testimonial: Weight Loss, Detoxification and Spiritual Benefits

Anna shared her remarkable experience with this practice. A practitioner of dry fasting for years, she recently completed a four-day dry fast, during which she consumed no food or water. As a result, she lost 4.5kg at the age of 39. In addition to the weight loss, Anna mentioned that she underwent detoxification and experienced spiritual benefits, mental breakthroughs and emotional cleansing. In a testimonial, she says: "I've been doing dry fasting for years and have just completed a four-day DRY FAST, which means no food or water (or anything). I lost ten pounds and went from 127 to 117 pounds at 39, detoxified, and experienced many spiritual benefits, mental breakthroughs and emotional cleansing."

Yvain Blechmans: Dry fasting has profoundly impacted me both physically and psychologically. It feels like a truly universal therapy without side effects, though it requires special attention and proper recovery. I was surprised by how much rest I needed, feeling fatigued even five days later. However, my body and mind have felt rejuvenated for a long time, thanks to Michel and Marie Christine.

Sébastien Pribetich: I would like to share my experience of dry fasting in July 2024. Unlike the other participants, my lifestyle was particularly unhealthy, living in Lille with excessive food and alcohol consumption. Previously, I had done dry fasting to manage these excesses, but my eating habits remained poor. I joined this retreat to learn how to exit fasting and eat healthily again.

To my great surprise, this cure offered much more than expected. Besides learning how to transition from fasting and re-feed healthily, I completely transformed my lifestyle. My diet is now balanced, and I no longer feel the urge to overeat. This experience has been a turning point, allowing me to rediscover a sense of well-being I never imagined possible.

Serge: I came to dry fasting retreat in Switzerland with Michel Deladoey as a preventive measure, without any existing pathologies, curious to experience the method developed by Michel and Marie Christine. On the advice of friends who spoke highly of it, I initially planned for five days but ended up doing six. I was surprised by the intensity of thirst and the profound state of grace I felt, experiencing extraordinary clarity and fluidity. Compared to water fasting, dry fasting is much more effective, providing intense cleansing and regeneration.

I experienced no violent elimination crises and enjoyed extraordinary mental clarity for a month afterward. My digestion and mental clarity improved, my nasal passages cleared, and I regained weight as I had been underweight. The gradual reintroduction of food in a supportive group setting was incredibly beneficial. This experience has been unparalleled, bringing about significant life changes and enhancing my overall well-being.

Alain: In 2021, I was diagnosed with prostate cancer. Prior to that, a friend introduced me to dry fasting, which turned out to be a profoundly different experience. My eight days of dry fasting retreat with Michel were emotionally intense but ultimately extraordinary, reinforcing my spiritual journey. The group dynamic was crucial, making fasting 60% more effective than doing it alone at home.

Also, your first book on dry fasting was enlightening and essential. This experience confirmed that dry fasting is a path I need to follow, and the group support and psycho-emotional assistance were invaluable. The gradual reintroduction of food was crucial for avoiding mistakes, and the modified state of consciousness post-fast was pleasantly sustained for weeks.

Georges: I embarked on a 7-day dry fast, preparing thoroughly for 1-2 months beforehand. The results were incredible. The group's support was instrumental in helping me through the process. I noticed significant improvements in my intestines, evacuating black sludge on the sixth day, which made me feel lighter and more energetic. My energy levels increased from 7.5 before retreat to 9.5 out of 10 two months after retreat.

This fast inspired me to make dietary changes and provided a great deal of mental calm. The entire experience, including the treatments and group interactions, was extraordinary. I highly recommend this cure to anyone and advise not overthinking it beforehand. Just go for it without fear.

Christian: At 65, suffering from bipolar disorder, I discovered dry fasting as a potential cure. The main difference compared to fasting alone was the gradual and successful reintroduction of food. Dry fasting allowed me to stop taking two medications, Ambipol and Seroquel, which had regulated my moods for ten years. This was incredible to me.

I did seven days of dry fasting and am considering going further next time. Fasting in a group boosted my self-confidence and improved the fasting experience. The connection to nature during the fast was profound. Compared to fasting alone at home, the group support and gradual return to eating were significant benefits. Montenegro, by the sea, is a magical place for this cure, and I plan to return.

About the author

Michel Deladoey, a Swiss naturopath, is a pioneer in the field of therapeutic dry fasting in Europe, but is also actively involved in research into the practice. His research efforts are aimed at deepening the scientific and holistic understanding of dry fasting since long times and exploring its potential health benefits. He is currently the only expert in Europe in this field with practical experience of accompanying fasters through this highly therapeutic process since 2010.

With a solid training in naturopathy from the College de Naturopathie Appliquée in Paris, supplemented by the Heilpraktiker examination and a State Diploma in Nutrition and Dietetics from the Faculty of Pharmacy in Clermont-Ferrand, France, he combines his skills in nutrition, micronutrition, energy medicines, hygiene and other holistic fields to enrich his practice and his research into dry fasting.

He has developed a unique method of dry fasting, combining emotional release therapies, yoga and naturopathy, and offers individual coaching and group retreats in Switzerland, Montenegro and Spain. His contribution to research in the field of therapeutic dry fasting reinforces his role as a leader and innovator in this specialist practice in the world.

Michel Deladoey is also the author of French book Therapeutic Dry Fasting, a book which reflects his expertise and in-depth knowledge. For more information about his unique approach, his services and his research work, you can visit his website www.jeunesec.com or visit him at his practice in Bex/VD, Switzerland.

Book presentation page

Dry fasting révolution Practical Guide, is a pioneering work which redefines the practice of fasting by shedding new light on it and providing previously unpublished data. This book is not just a theoretical exploration; it is the fruit of real-life experience, bearing witness to the remarkable effectiveness of dry fasting in supporting patients undergoing treatment.

Discover a revolutionary approach to dry fasting that is more effective than other types of fasting. Through total abstinence from food and water, this method triggers unprecedented deep healing and cellular regeneration. This book reveals recent scientific data and captivating testimonials, illustrating how dry fasting can transform physical, mental and emotional health.

Drawing on his experience of supporting patients undergoing dry fasting, the author shares practical advice and proven strategies for a safe and successful fasting experience. Explore unique techniques for preparing the body and mind for fasting, managing the detoxification phases, and gradually reintegrating a healthy post-fasting diet.

This book is an indispensable guide for those seeking to explore the depths of this ancient practice, reinvented for holistic effectiveness and transformation. Embark on this adventure of health and self-discovery, and enjoy an unforgettable dry fasting experience.

Visit the website www.jeunesec.com to find out about upcoming dates, treatments, appointments for consultations and products on sale.
Retreat : https://www.jeunesec.com/prochaines-dates.html
Retreat VIP one to three people in the place of your choice.
email :Michel.deladoey@gmail.com

Online therapeutic dry fasting training to do at home in French only:
https://formations.jeunesec.com/bdc-jeune-sec-therapeutique/

Michel's previous book: *Le jeûne sec thérapeutique (Therapeutic dry fasting)* https://www.editionsmarcopietteur.com/testez/345-le-jeune-sec-therapeutique-9782874611421.html

Michel Deladoey, naturopath and therapeutic dry fasting coach/ consultation FR/EN
www.jeunesec.com
+41794367152
Michel.deladoey@gmail.com

Bibliography

- Deladoey M. (2020). Therapeutic dry fasting. Éditions Marco Pietteur
- Filonov S. (2008). *Dry fasting, myths and reality.*
- Shelton H. (1996). Fasting and health? *Courrier du Livre.*
- Souren A. A. (1994). *Will we live to be three hundred?* N ° 6.
- Souvorin A. A. (1998). *Souvorin's method. Fasting treatment.*
- Vassioutin A. (2010). *Esprit tout-puissant or simple and effective self-healing techniques.*

Scientific references – English-language research articles

1. World Health Organization (WHO) (2010). Global recommendations on physical activity for health. Geneva, Switzerland: WHO.

2. Swift, D.L., McGee, J.E., et al. 2018). The effects of exercise and physical activity on weight loss and maintenance. Progress in cardiovascular diseases, 61(2), pp.206-213.

3 Warburton, D.E. and Bredin, S.S., (2017). Health benefits of physical activity: a systematic review of current systematic reviews. Current opinion in cardiology, 32(5), pp.541-556.

4. World Cancer Research Fund/American Institute for Cancer Research. Continuous Update Project Expert Report (2018). Physical activity and the risk of cancer.

5. Cruz-Jentoft AJ, Sayer AA (2019). Sarcopenia. The Lancet. 393 (10191): 2636-2646.

6. Stubbs, B., Vancampfort, D. et al, (2018). EPA guidance on physical activity as a treatment for severe mental illness: a meta-review of the evidence and Position Statement from EPA, supported by OPTMH. European Psychiatry, 54, pp.124-144.

7. Tari, A.R., Norevik, C.S., et al. (2019). Are the neuroprotective effects of exercise training systemically mediated? Progress in cardiovascular diseases.

8. Livingston, G., Sommerlad, A., et al. (2017). Dementia prevention, intervention, and care. The Lancet, 390(10113), 2673-2734.

Made in United States
Orlando, FL
12 February 2025